OXFORD MEDICAL PUBLICATIONS

Emergencies in Palliative and Supportive Care

Emergencies in Palliative and Supportive Care

David Currow

Chair, Department of Palliative and Supportive Services,
Flinders University, Adelaide, Australia

Director, Southern Adelaide Palliative Services,
Daw Park, Adelaide, Australia

Director, International Institute of Palliative & Supportive
Studies, Adelaide, Australia

Katherine Clark

Senior Staff Specialist, Royal Prince Alfred Hospital,
Camperdown, Sydney, Australia

Clinical Senior Lecturer, University of Sydney,
Sydney, Australia

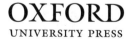

OXFORD
UNIVERSITY PRESS

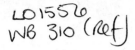

OXFORD
UNIVERSITY PRESS

Great Clarendon Street, Oxford OX2 6DP

Oxford University Press is a department of the University of Oxford.
It furthers the University's objective of excellence in research, scholarship,
and education by publishing worldwide in

Oxford New York

Auckland Cape Town Dar es Salaam Hong Kong Karachi
Kuala Lumpur Madrid Melbourne Mexico City Nairobi
New Delhi Shanghai Taipei Toronto

With offices in

Argentina Austria Brazil Chile Czech Republic France Greece
Guatemala Hungary Italy Japan Poland Portugal Singapore
South Korea Switzerland Thailand Turkey Ukraine Vietnam

Oxford is a registered trade mark of Oxford University Press
in the UK and in certain other countries

Published in the United States
by Oxford University Press Inc., New York

British Library Cataloguing in Publication Data
Data available

Library of Congress Cataloging in Publication Data
Data available

Typeset by Newgen Imaging Systems (P) Ltd., Chennai, India
Printed in Italy
on acid-free paper by
Legoprint S.p.A

ISBN 0–19–856722–7 (Flexicover: alk.paper)

  978–0–19–856722–6 (Flexicover: alk.paper)

'… give us strength:

strength to hang on,

strength to let go.'

Michael Leunig
The Common Prayer Collection
Penguin 1990

'Quick! I'm not dead yet…'
Anon

Acute-on-chronic dyspnoea
- **Pleural effusions** (p.268) and **pericardial effusions** (p.100) often have an insidious onset with progressive breathlessness that worsens from occurring on significant exertion to occurring at rest.
- **A cancer associated with lymphangitis carcinomatosis** (p.284): often in a person with primary breast cancer.
- **Worsening cachexia**: in all end-stage illness breathlessness will worsen as death approaches.
- **Increasing ascites** reduces diaphragmatic excursion (p.144)
- **A history of bleomycin use** often has an insidious onset.
- **A history cardiomyopathy** often has a gradual onset.
- **A history of chronic airways disease**: check for sputum production, fever, wheezing (p.278). Consider an infective exacerbation. These people may have been smokers. If this is associated with weight loss and increasing fatigue, consider the development of primary lung cancers.

Can you modify anything contributing to the symptom?

Thromboembolism is treatable with the aim of reducing the incidence of fatal pulmonary emboli (p.106).

Community-acquired pneumonia in the presence of no other significant lung pathology and a functioning immune system can be treated (p.264).

People with **lymphangitis carcinomatosis** should be treated symptomatically (p.284).

For an **acute myocardial infarction**, further myocardial damage can be minimized (p.110). (Use of thrombolytics is limited to people with no recent GIT bleeding and no intracerebral pathology.)

Unloculated **pleural effusions** can be treated with pleural drainage and ideally with pleurodesis (p.268).

Fluid overload can be improved in most people except in end-stage disease and hypoalbuminaemia (p.110).

Pericardial effusions can be drained, affording significant relief (p.100).

Increasing abdominal girth due to **ascites** can be quickly relieved by peritoneal tap. The addition of diuretics may also be effective (p.144).

People who present with worsening **heart failure** may improve by ensuring that anaemia is reversed and any associated infections are treated. Ensure that management of heart failure has been maximized (p.110).

People with **anaemia** may be transfused. Consider the burden of this intervention in very late stage illness.

An **infective exacerbation of airways disease** warrants antibiotics, corticosteroids, and possibly bronchodilators. (p.278).

What underlying factors cannot be improved?

Cachexia without an ability to reverse the underlying catabolic state will progress. Late **drug toxicity** is irreversible and often progresses. Although **loculated pleural effusions** can be treated with videoscopically assisted thoracentesis, the procedure is limited to people who have a good functional status.

Symptomatic treatment

Non-pharmacological intervention

There are good data to support energy conservation (in conjunction with an occupational therapist) and relaxation/visualization techniques to minimize breathlessness.

Avoid unnecessary exercise.

People's sense of impending doom is often overwhelming as breathlessness tends to worsen as the disease progresses. The need to address these understandable fears is central to the support of a person at the end-of-life.

Pharmacological intervention

Regular low-dose oral morphine (20 mg per 24 hs or 10 mg parenterally every 24 hs) in opioid-naïve people with refractory breathlessness will help relieve dyspnoea. An increase of 30–50 per cent per dose may be necessary in people already on opioids.

A regular dose of an anxiolytic such as a long-acting benzodiazepine (clonazepam 0.5 mg twice daily or lorazepam 0.5–1.0 mg SL twice daily) may have a role late in disease.

Oxygen may be of benefit in people who are hypoxaemic. Flowing air may be of significant benefit in people with normal oxygen tension.

Any person with a wheeze should have a trial of a bronchodilator (salbutamol 2.5–5.0 mg nebulized four times daily, ipratropium bromide 250–500 µg nebulized four times daily, 0.9 per cent NaCl 5 ml nebulized as required).

A person with stridor or lymphangitis may have a trial of oral dexamethasone 4–8 mg in the morning.

With noisy terminal respiratory secretions, subcutaneous hyoscine butylbromide 20 mg SC every 4 hs may be of limited symptomatic benefit.

Further reading

Oxford Textbook of Medicine, Vol. 3, pp. 1403–1404.
Oxford Textbook of Palliative Medicine, p. 922.
Oxford Handbook of Palliative Care, pp. 296–299.

Acute confusional state (delirium)

Onset of symptom

Delirium is characterized by a fluctuating mental state. Even late in disease, people value clear mentation (p.208).

Acute onset (less than 24 hs) of confusion and ...

- **Recent new medications** can add to the existing anticholinergic load from long-term medications and cause an acute delirium.
- **Recently commenced corticosteroids** may precipitate an agitated delirium.
- **Asterixis**: metabolic factors including severe uraemia (totally obstructed renal tract) (p.292) or hepatic decompensation (p.154) especially with upper GIT bleeding may precipitate a delirium.
- **Hypoxaemia** (p.24) can cause acute confusion. (Be concerned about the introduction of oxygen for breathlessness in a person with a history of carbon dioxide retention; this can cause respiratory depression in a small number of susceptible people with central hypoventilation states).
- **Sepsis**: acute sepsis can include community-acquired pneumonia (p.264), biliary tract sepsis (p.148), meningitis (p.216), or a urinary tract infection (p.290) (especially in the elderly).
- **Atrial fibrillation or mechanical heart valve**: consider a transient ischaemic event or stroke (p.208).
- **Recent admission to hospital** may cause delirium in a person with an underlying dementia.
- Known past history of cerebral metastases, or past history of CVA should prompt consideration of **seizures** (p.210).

Subacute onset (1–3 days) of confusion

- **Recent medication withdrawal** (including benzodiazepines, glucocorticoids, tobacco, alcohol, or SSRIs).
- **Febrile or hypotensive**: sepsis often causes a subtle onset of confusion, urinary tract infection, atypical pneumonia, or cellulitis.
- **Continued use of antihypertensives** late into the course of a life-limiting illness can cause cerebral hypoperfusion.
- **Ascites**: consider spontaneous bacterial peritonitis (p.144).
- **Dehydration** may be a significant contributor with increased insensible losses (air conditioning, hot weather), decreased oral intake, or high output states (ileostomies, fistulae (p.158).
- **Metabolic derangements**: the onset masks a much longer time course over which **hypercalcaemia** (p.260) or **hyponatraemia** (p.194) develop. (Exclude diuretics as a cause for hyponatraemia).
- **Hypoglycaemia** is rarely seen unless the person is taking hypoglycaemic agents (p.248).
- **Cerebral metastases** may directly contribute to confusion depending where the lesions are. (This includes meningeal disease). CNS disease of any aetiology may cause **hyponatraemia** with SIADH (p.196).
- Recent radiological investigations with contrast may precipitate **hyperthyroidism** in some people (p.256).

- **In the terminal phase of a life-limiting illness**: acute confusional states are frequently encountered towards death. If the deterioration is expected, treat symptomatically. If it is unexpected and appears to precipitate the terminal phase, consider the other differential diagnoses.

Acute-on-chronic confusion
- A clear differential diagnosis needs to be drawn from **dementia**. Many people with subtle dementia may be found to have short-term memory problems for the first time as the catabolic insult of advanced disease unmasks a previously unrecognized dementia.
- **Untreated depression and anxiety** may present with features of delirium (p.238 & p.242).
- **Progressive cachexia** may contribute to a susceptibility to delirium independent of identifiable nutritional deficiencies.
- **A history of alcohol misuse**: always have a low threshold for the introduction of thiamine until the cause for confusion becomes established.

Can you modify anything contributing to the symptom?

There is often a lag of days between reducing or reversing precipitating causes of delirium and seeing cognition improve.

All medications need to be reviewed. The newest medications (often opioids) may be adding to an anticholinergic load precipitating an acute confusional state. It may be possible to reduce long-term medications in order to reduce the anticholinergic load while continuing the opioids.

Sepsis can be treated and this may be one of the most important aspects of reducing acute confusion. Recurrent sepsis or sepsis in the setting of severe immunocompromise or prolonged neutropaenia may become untreatable.

Hepatic decompensation is often amenable to treatment; stop any GIT bleeding, use lactulose or neomycin to decrease gut transit time, and minimize protein intake until mentation improves (p.154).

Dehydration can be treated with the judicious use of parenteral hydration. In the terminal phases of a life-limiting illness, hydration needs are not great and small amounts of fluid are all that is necessary; larger volumes are likely to cause peripheral or pulmonary oedema and increased GIT secretions.

Hypercalcaemia may respond to bisphosphonates (p.260). Where low serum sodium is secondary to SIADH, fluid restriction may be of benefit (although most people in this setting already have low fluid intakes).

Resetting **glycaemic control** (8–14 mmol/l) is likely to reverse problems associated with hypoglycaemia (p.248).

Newly diagnosed **cerebral metastases** may improve with the addition of oral dexamethasone (4–8 mg daily).

Treat **hypoxaemia** with oxygen. Consider the person's past history of airways disease. In people who are well enough, collect arterial blood gases to guide oxygen flow rates.

Seizures may cause delirium in the post-ictal phase or in the presence of status epilepticus. Attempts to arrest seizure activity should be made with prompt administration of benzodiazepines and antiseizure medications (p.210).

What underlying factors cannot be improved?

Without an ability to reverse the underlying systemic illness, **cachexia** cannot be reversed. Often, despite attempts, reversing metabolic factors late in illness does not improve cognition.

Despite therapeutic advances, **dementia** is not yet amenable to treatment late in the course of a life-limiting illness.

Symptomatic treatment

Non-pharmacological intervention

Disorientation is frightening to people; the sensations of hallucinations are real and often overwhelming. A quiet, familiar environment with prompts that orientate a person to time and place helps. Family and staff sensitivity to acute confusion is crucial.

If this is occurring at the end-of-life, consider whether or not constipation, acute retention of urine, or pain due to uncomfortable positioning may be contributing to this state.

Pharmacological intervention

Acute confusional states need to be treated actively. Antipsychotics (haloperidol 0.5–3.0 mg orally or SC daily, risperidone 0.5–1.0 mg daily or twice daily, olanzapine 2.5–5.0 mg daily, chlorpromazine 25–50 mg orally or SC once to three times daily) should be titrated to response with regular doses. Haloperidol and chlorpromazine can have extrapyramidal effects, especially in the frail and elderly. Chlorpromazine may be more sedating at the same antipsychotic dose.

At times, in severe confusional states not responding to antipsychotics, sedation should be offered with long-acting benzodiazepines such as diazepam 2–5 mg once to three times daily or lorazepam 0.5–1.0 mg SL once to four times daily in doses sufficient to ensure that the amnesic effects of benzodiazepines are not worsening the confusion.

Further reading

Oxford Textbook of Medicine, Vol. 3, pp. 1274–1275, 1283–1284, 1405–1407.
Oxford Textbook of Palliative Medicine, pp. 708–713.
Oxford Handbook of Palliative Care, pp. 432–436.

Decreased level of consciousness

Onset of symptom

Acute onset (less than 24 hs) of decreased level of consciousness and...

- **A history of falls, anticoagulation, or coagulopathy**: subarachnoid bleed is an urgent diagnosis of exclusion (p.220).
- **A CNS tumour**: consider raised intracranial pressure (p.224) (with hydrocephalus, intracranial bleed or coning), or seizures (p.210).
- **New medications**: consider medications with sedating effects including opioids, benzodiazepines, tricyclic antidepressants, or anticonvulsants (e.g. phenytoin has non-linear pharmacokinetics)(p.58).
- **Recent changes in medication doses**: decrease in glucocorticoids, Addisonian crisis in people on long-term glucocorticoids (p.254), failure to take thyroid replacement (p.258), or recent increase in opioids, sedatives, antidepressants, anticonvulsants, or antiemetics.
- **Fever**: sources of infection including meningitis (p.216), encephalitis (including primary herpetic infections in the immunocompromised), or renal/respiratory tract sepsis (pp.264, 268) causing systemic shut-down. People on long-term glucocorticoids who become septic need to have urgent adrenal replacement.
- **History of diabetes**: Consider hypoglycaemia especially if oral intake is variable and hypoglycaemic agents have continued without dose revision (p.248). Also consider hyperglycaemia (p.250) (ketoacidosis, hyperosmolar coma) as a cause of an acute deterioration.
- **Oxygen therapy**: carbon dioxide retention may cause a decreased level of consciousness as CO_2 levels rise.

Subacute onset (1–3 days) of decreased levels of consciousness and...

- **Severe hepatic dysfunction**: hepatic encephalopathy can cause progressive obtundation (p.154).
- **Anuria or decreased urinary output**: pre-renal causes include dehydration, renal causes are often associated with drug toxicity, and post-renal causes include obstruction of the urinary tract (intraluminal, extraluminal) (p.292).
- **Dehydration**: people who continue with decreased oral intake may have severe pre-renal impairment. High output stomas or fistulae, especially involving the small bowel, can rapidly lead to dehydration if oral intake is not sufficient.
- **History of diminishing function** consistent with an expected death as the body closes down from a life-limiting illness.
- **Space-occupying lesion**: consider complex partial seizures in the differential diagnosis (p.210).
- **Vascular disease or atrial fibrillation**: consider transient ischaemic attack or stroke as a cause.
- In a person with known mediastinal disease consider **superior vena cava obstruction** where the first presentation may be with obtundation (p.94).

- In a person with cancer (solid/haematological) this may be a presentation of **hypercalcaemia** (p.260). Consider other paraneoplastic phenomena such as SIADH (p.196), cerebellar degeneration, and encephalitis.

Acute-on-chronic changes in level of consciousness
- **History of frailty and dementia**: consider **subdural haematoma** (p.220) although a history of falls or head trauma may not be forthcoming.
- **History of a space-occupying lesion**: increase in the size of the lesion may lead to diminishing consciousness.

Can you modify anything contributing to the symptom?

Subdural bleeds need to be treated in people where contributing pathology, such as coagulopathy, can be reversed. Intracranial and subarachnoid bleeds are likely to have much worse outcomes in this population.

Medications (new medications, medications with recent dose changes, and medications that may accumulate) need to be reviewed carefully. Non-prescribed medications or people who have had several professionals writing prescriptions need to have thorough histories taken. The history of transdermal medications may be forgotten in people with a decreased level of consciousness.

Sepsis can generally be treated.

Obstructive hydrocephalus needs neurosurgical review especially if the person has otherwise being functioning well.

Epilepsy (p.210) can be treated, and if it is the cause of changed consciousness or mentation this is likely to improve the person's function considerably.

Dehydration contributing directly to decreased levels of consciousness can be treated with the judicious use of parenteral hydration. In the absence of identifiable causes of decreased level of consciousness, hydration alone is unlikely to make a substantial difference.

Hyponatraemia is amenable to therapy in someone who is functioning reasonably well (p.194).

Carbon dioxide retention should be treated with a decrease in supplemental oxygen and optimizing respiratory function.

Hypercalcaemia (p.260), especially at first presentation, is usually reversible with bisphosphonates and gentle hydration.

Hypoglycaemia (p.248) and **hyperglycaemia** (p.250) can be corrected.

What underlying factors cannot be improved?

Without an ability to reverse the underlying catabolic state, **cachexia** cannot be reversed.

Intracranial and **subarachnoid bleeds,** especially in late-stage disease, are not likely to be operable given the overall circumstances of the person.

Symptomatic treatment

Non-pharmacological intervention

A calm peaceful environment is important. Even though people with a decreased level of consciousness may not be able to respond, there are data that demonstrate that they can still hear familiar voices and feel familiar touch. Supporting families to continue to spend time and have conversations with the person is important.

In a person with impaired consciousness, speech therapist review of swallowing may lessen difficulties with oral intake or medications being aspirated. People with impaired consciousness should not take anything by mouth until this assessment is done.

Pharmacological intervention

If the person has already been on symptom control medications, these should be continued by an appropriate route of administration (sub-lingual, rectal, transdermal or subcutaneous).

Further reading

Oxford Textbook of Medicine, Vol. 3, pp. 988–992.
Oxford Handbook of Palliative Care, pp. 381–385.

Agitation

Onset of symptom

Acute onset (less than 24 hs) of agitation

- **Unrelieved physical symptoms** especially pain and nausea, urinary retention, or constipation.
- **History of a psychiatric disorder**: delirium, agitated depression, or hypomania can all present as agitation.
- **Recent bad news**: the person with the life-limiting illness may have had bad news or the immediacy of dying may have started to have an impact in a very specific way. Fears which are often difficult to articulate, anxiety, frustration, or recurrent nightmares may all contribute to agitation. Previous experience of other people close to them in life dying may influence how they see their own death.
- **Medications known to cause agitation** including drugs with dopaminergic effects that can cause akathisia (including metoclopramide and haloperidol) or those which may occasionally cause paradoxical agitation such as opioids and benzodiazepines.
- **Acute confusional state**, with any of its causes (p.28).
- **Impaired ability to communicate**: unable to verbalize, especially in the setting of an expressive or receptive aphasia.
- **Hypoxaemia** (p.24).

Subacute onset (1–3 days) of agitation

- **Fevers, hypothermia, or hypotension**: sepsis can present as agitation, especially occult urinary (p.290) or respiratory tract infections (p.264).

Acute-on-chronic anxiety

With a history of anxiety: **anxiety states** (p.242) may cause agitation and be exacerbated by evidence of disease progression or loss of function. **Depression** (p.238) and anxiety often coexist. **Adjustment disorders** may also have a component of agitation. Long-term **schizophrenia** may have an element of low-grade agitation.

Can you modify anything contributing to the symptom?

An open discussion about the agitation is a key issue. Eliciting fears in a supportive way while respecting how difficult it is to talk about many of these issues, may be very helpful.

Medications causing extrapyramidal side-effects can usually be stopped or a substitute found. For example, domperidone can be substituted for metoclopramide for nausea because domperidone does not cross the blood–brain barrier.

Acute psychiatric problems need adequate assessment. Even late in the course of illness, treating psychiatric problems is important. In someone acutely depressed, assess risk for suicide (p.240). (Does the person wish to hasten death? Has the person thought about how they would end their life? Has the person ever attempted suicide before? Have they made actual plans to end their life? What support do they have from family, friends or health professionals? Are they depressed?)

What underlying factors cannot be improved?

Often there are limited choices in replacing or withdrawing key medications that are maintaining function or comfort.

Symptomatic treatment

Non-pharmacological intervention

What does this person think is causing their agitation? Do they have insight into the agitation and its possible causes?

Pharmacological intervention

There is a place for the short-term use of appropriate anxiolytics. This may include a benzodiazepine such as lorazepam.

SSRIs have a specific role to play in panic attacks. This may be while underlying causes of the agitation are reversed or in the clinical setting where no reversible causes are found.

Restless legs, independent of the factors already outlined, can be an entity in themselves, worse at night and very distressing. Treatment should include:

- stop excess intake of stimulants
- replace electrolyte and vitamin deficiancies
- consider a trial of dopaminergic agents (bromocriptine, pergolide), or in mild cases, benzodiazepines (clonazepam).

Further reading

Oxford textbook of medicine, Vol. 3, pp.1283–1286, 1405.
Oxford Handbook of Palliative Care, pp. 744–745.

Diarrhoea

Onset of symptom

Secretory (compared with non-secretory diarrhoea) persists even with fasting. Secretory diarrhoea is characterized by high-volume, watery diarrhoea. Causes include *Vibrio cholerae* and *Escherichia coli*, *Shigella*, *Campylobacter* species and viral infections, medications (methylxanthines), and hormone-secreting tumours (serotonin, calcitonin, gastrin, and vasoactive intestinal peptide).

Acute onset (less than 24 hs) of diarrhoea

- **Influenza-like symptoms**: viral gastroenteritis is the most common cause of acute diarrhoea. Other infectious agents include *Giardia lamblia* and *Clostridium difficile*, especially with a recent history of antibiotics causing pseudo-membranous colitis (p.130). Any antibiotic in the previous 4 weeks is implicated, but it is particularly associated with ampicillin, amoxicillin and cephalosporins.

Subacute onset (1–3 days) of diarrhoea

- **Recent radiotherapy** (involving bowel directly in the field of therapy) can present with increasing severity of diarrhoea (p.130).
- **Recent chemotherapy,** especially with 5-fluorouracil, methotrexate, or doxorubicin.
- Over-zealous use of **aperients** (probably the most common cause) and other medications (antibiotics, NSAIDs, antacids, glutamate).
- **Colonic and rectal tumours.**
- **Enterocolonic fistula** (p.158) in a person with known malignancies, past history of surgery, or radiotherapy.

Acute-on-chronic diarrhoea

- **History of constipation** with faecal overflow.
- **History of inflammatory bowel disease (IBD)**: consider whether people are not tolerating routine medications for IBD, such as people with uncontrolled vomiting or late-stage anorexia (p.130).
- **History of pancreatic disease** with steatorrhoea.
- **Previous GIT surgery** with short bowel or blind loop syndrome or bile salt diarrhoea because of a previous ileal resection.
- **History of diabetes mellitus** with autonomic neuropathy.
- **Thyroid replacement** therapy that has not been adjusted as the person loses weight.
- **Neuroendocrine tumours including carcinoid** (especially towards the end of the dose for long-acting octreotide).
- **AIDS** from organisms including cryptosporidium, *Mycoplasma avium intracellulare* (MAI), *Giardia lamblia*, cytomegalovirus, or herpes simplex virus.

Can you modify anything contributing to the symptom?

Hydration status should be assessed and corrected.

Viral gastroenteritis requires support; for most people oral rehydration should be sufficient. Rarely, specific electrolyte problems will need parenteral support.

Check recent use of **antibiotics** (*Clostridium difficile* toxin can be identified in stools and treated with oral vancomycin 125 mg every 6 hs. Resolution of symptoms is expected within the first 2 days). Check for recent overseas travel.

Exclude **constipation** with faecal overflow with a plain abdominal X-ray looking for faecal loading.

In **pancreatic insufficiency**, use pancreatic enzyme replacement with food.

People with **ileal resection** may benefit from cholestyramine (4 g three times daily).

Corticosteroids and mesalazine (500 mg orally three times daily) should be used to treat **inflammatory bowel disease**.

Chemotherapy may be of significant benefit in managing neuro-endocrine tumours.

Regular octreotide (100 μg SC three times daily) may be of benefit in people with **radiation-induced diarrhoea** to reduce fluid loss and the length of any hospital admission.

Review current medications used for **constipation** and reduce if necessary.

What underlying factors cannot be improved?

In shortened bowel (surgery, fistula formation), controlling long-term frequent loose bowel motions can be difficult. Failure to do so may lead to numerous adverse consequences, including dehydration, malnutrition, electrolyte imbalance, and impaired immune function.

Symptomatic treatment

Non-pharmacological intervention

Fluid support is the mainstay of non-pharmacological intervention. Bulking agents such as ispaghula husks can be of benefit to decrease frequency of diarrhoea and improve continence control.

Pharmacological intervention

Identify infective causes and treat vigorously even late in the course of a life-limiting illness.

Opioids (morphine 5 mg orally or 2.5 mg SC, as required/every 4 hs) can be used for diarrhoea.

Oral cholestyramine (4 g three times daily) can be used to manage diarrhoea secondary to shortened ileum.

Octreotide (start with 100 μg three times daily) may be of use in truly refractory diarrhoea (*Cryptosporidium*, carcinoid, Zollinger–Ellison syndrome, high-output ileostomy).

Add 5-HT$_3$ antagonists (ondansetron 4 mg SL/IV/SC) in Zollinger–Ellison syndrome.

Further reading

Oxford Textbook of Medicine, Vol. 2 pp. 311, 488–489, 574, 663–665.
Oxford Textbook of Palliative Medicine, pp. 483–93, 864.
Oxford Handbook of Palliative Care, pp. 258–259.

Nausea (and vomiting)

Be sure that this person has nausea rather than anorexia. The concepts are often used interchangeably by patients.

Nausea is the unpleasant sensation of wanting to vomit. It is a distressing and feared complication of illness.

Onset of symptom

Acute onset (less than 24 hs) of nausea

- **A history of new medications including recent chemotherapy**.
  Review new medications but always consider that the new medication, may be crucial to symptom control and other medications with which they may be interacting can be stopped. Medications often blamed include opioids, antibiotics, cytotoxic agents, digoxin, and iron supplements. Always ask about non-prescribed medications, including complementary or alternative products.
- **Epigastric discomfort**: consider gastritis, peptic ulcer disease, gastric outlet obstruction, and intestinal obstruction. Gastritis is more common with NSAIDs or NSAIDs used in combination with glucocorticoids, or recent upper abdominal radiotherapy.
- **Known cerebral metastases**: consider an acute increase in intracranial pressure including acute intracranial bleed (p.220), ventricular obstruction causing acute hydrocephalus, or a rise in pressure due to tumour progression. Nausea can occur with any leptomeningeal malignant infiltration or cerebellar metastases.
- **Fever, rigors, hypotension, or hypothermia**: consider sepsis as a cause for acute onset nausea. Occult sites include the urinary tract (especially with the presence of hydronephrosis) (p.288), cholecystitis (p.148), or atypical chest infections (p.264).
- **Unrelieved pain** may lead to nausea.

Sub-acute onset (1–3 days) of nausea

- **Nausea associated with movement**. Consider cerebellar metastases, irritation of the vestibular apparatus, or gastroparesis (secondary to opioids or ascites).
- **Worsening renal failure** renal impairment can both present as worsening nausea. Consider ureteric obstruction (p.288) as an acute worsening for renal failure or medication toxicity (aminoglycosides or anti-inflammatory agents).
- **Worsening hepatic failure**: hepatic impairment can present as worsening nausea. Consider drug toxicity (excessive ingestion of paracetamol) or Budd–Chiari syndrome (hepatic vein thrombosis) for hepatic failure (p.154).
- **Evidence of sepsis**: consider less typical sites if there is clear evidence of sepsis and no obvious site (endocarditis infective (p.104), non-bacterial meningitis, or abscess formation including a cerebral abscess). The elderly and immunocompromised will often have less florid presentations of sepsis.
- **Anxiety and fear**.

- **Electrolyte abnormalities** (hypercalcaemia (p.260), hyponatraemia (p.194) may also be associated with nausea.
- **Gastric compression** associated with hepatomegaly, ascites, or peritoneal disease may cause nausea and early satiety.

Acute-on-chronic nausea
- **Any of the causes of nausea already mentioned**: all of these causes can have a more protracted onset with acute worsening.
- **Eating:** (often at the insistence of well-meaning family and friends) despite anorexia as part of the cachexia syndrome.
- **Cerebral disease.**
- **Anxiety**: the diagnosis of anticipatory nausea, or fear and anxiety causing nausea, is one of exclusion but should be considered in the overall assessment in people with refractory symptoms.
- **Constipation**: should not by itself cause vomiting. However, it can cause significant nausea which worsens with the constipation.

Can you modify anything contributing to the symptom?
Advice about not eating when the person is not hungry is crucial to controlling nausea for many people with advanced disease.

Medications contributing directly to nausea (e.g. antibiotics) or specific toxicity (e.g. anti-inflammatories causing gastritis) should be stopped or a substitution made with an agent that will cause less nausea.

Reducing cerebral oedema for any cause of raised intracranial pressure is important. Use of glucocorticoids (oral dexamethasone 8 mg in the morning and at mid-day) may help to reduce cerebral oedema while the underlying exacerbating causes are defined. Gastric irritation should be treated expectantly with a PPI or H_2 receptor antagonist.

Drainage of tense ascites may reduce nausea and allow oral intake.

What underlying factors cannot be improved?
As nausea is often a manifestation of the underlying disease state, without an ability to change the course of the life-limiting illness, a predominantly symptomatic approach is needed. People with leptomeningeal spread of cancer or rapidly worsening renal function often have refractory nausea.

Symptomatic treatment
Non-pharmacological intervention
Many people with nausea at the end-of-life have heightened sensitivity to smell, linked with substantial changes in tastes. Ensuring minimal exposure to the smell of food cooking is important.

Refocusing oral intake on preferred foods, in preferred amounts at preferred times (rather than a 'balanced' diet where people eat in volumes, at times and types of food that they do not feel like) is a key management strategy.

Check hydration status (tissue turgor, presence of tachycardia or hypotension) and carefully reverse any deficit.

Pharmacological intervention

Choices of medications to treat nausea are not well linked to the likely pathophysiology.

Initiate antiemetics based on the pattern of nausea and/or vomiting.

Metabolic causes of nausea may respond to haloperidol (0.5–3.0 mg orally or SC at night regularly).

CNS causes may respond to dexamethasone (4–8 mg orally or SC daily).

Evidence of gastroparesis should be treated with metoclopramide (10 mg orally or SC four times daily). (If there is any suspicion of GIT obstruction, pro-peristaltic agents such as metoclopramide or domperidone should be avoided. Aperients should also be stopped completely in suspected GIT obstruction.)

Cytotoxic-induced nausea and vomiting should be pre-emptively and managed with antiemetics prior to treatment (dexamethasone 4–8 mg immediately, lorazepam 0.5–1.0 mg SL immediately), during treatment (5-HT$_3$ antagonists/dexamethasone, aprepitant (selective NK-1 antagonist), metoclopramide), and after therapy (dexamethasone, metoclopramide).

Medications such as chlorpromazine or levopromeprazine may be useful in people with refractory nausea.

Further reading

Oxford Textbook of Medicine, Vol. 2, p. 488; Vol. 3, pp. 1401–1402.
Oxford Textbook of Palliative Medicine, pp. 459–466.
Oxford Handbook of Palliative Care, pp. 246–253.

Unheralded vomiting

Onset of symptom

Vomiting is the forceful expulsion of the gastric contents through the mouth. It is unpleasant and feared.

Acute onset (less than 24 hs) of vomiting

- **History of new medications**: check that new pro-peristaltic agents (metoclopramide or domperidone, sennosides) have not been added in someone with the potential of a bowel obstruction (p.140).
- **Epigastric discomfort**: consider pre-pyloric ulceration secondary to anti-inflammatories or glucocorticoids (especially if the person is on both).
- **Known cerebral metastases or leptomeningeal disease**: consider an acute increase in intracranial pressure including acute intracranial bleed, ventricular obstruction causing acute hydrocephalus, or a rise in pressure due to tumour progression. There is often no preceding nausea, and vomiting can occur at any time.
- **Bowel obstruction**: the more proximal the bowel obstruction, the more likely the person is to have unheralded vomiting. The obstruction does not need to be a total obstruction and so the person may still be passing flatus and stool (p.140).

Subacute onset (1–3 days) of unheralded vomiting

- **Nausea associated with movement**: consider cerebellar metastases or irritation of the vestibular apparatus.
- **Ascites or gross hepatomegaly**: squashed stomach can lead to unheralded vomiting that worsens as the pressure crushing the stomach worsens (p.144).

Can you modify anything contributing to the symptom?

In upper GIT obstruction, advice about small volumes of clear fluids frequently is crucial to minimising vomiting for many people with advanced disease. The volume of gastric secretions can be reduced using a H_2 receptor antagonist (ranitidine 300 mg orally twice daily or 50 mg SC four times daily). PPIs do not reduce the volume of upper GIT secretions).

Reducing cerebral oedema with any cause of raised intracranial pressure is important. Use of glucocorticoids (oral dexamethasone 8 mg in the morning and at mid-day) may help to reduce cerebral oedema while the underlying exacerbating causes are defined.

In someone who is not cachectic, consider other methods of providing nutrition if vomiting is only related to inoperable obstructions.

With raised intracranial pressure, exclude an undiagnosed subdural haematoma. With cerebral metastases, consider dexamethasone and whole brain radiotherapy. With obstructive hydrocephalus in someone who is otherwise well, consider a neurosurgical opinion for the insertion of a VP shunt.

What underlying factors cannot be improved?

Bowel obstruction, especially multilevel obstruction from malignant peritoneal seeding, will not be amenable to stenting, surgical bypass, or a defunctioning ileostomy.

A squashed stomach will continue to be symptomatic for most people.

Symptomatic treatment

Non-pharmacological intervention

Oral intake for squashed stomach relies on changing oral intake to small frequent snacks.

In bowel obstruction, oral fluids will continue to be tolerated unless the obstruction includes the jejunum, duodenum, or stomach.

Pharmacological intervention

If there is any suspicion of GIT obstruction, pro-peristaltic agents such as metoclopramide or domperidone should be avoided. Aperients should also be stopped completely in suspected GIT obstruction.

In addition to regular ranitidine, hyoscine butylbromide 20 mg SC every 4 hs regularly is likely to help with any colicky pain.

If an obstruction is not settling, octreotide 100–200 µg SC three times daily regularly may help to reduce frequency and volume of vomiting.

Further reading

Oxford Textbook of Medicine, Vol. 2, pp. 488, 1255.
Oxford Handbook of Palliative Care, pp. 246–253, 262–263.

Fever

Symptoms of sepsis with a very acute onset are much more likely to be either bacterial or viral infections.

In people with progressive life-limiting illnesses, the elderly, and those on long-term immunosuppression (including glucocorticoids), signs of sepsis may be muted.

Fever may also be due to non-infectious causes.

Onset of symptom

Acute onset (less than 24 hs) of fever and...

- **Recent cytotoxic chemotherapy**: although some agents are less likely to cause neutropenia, check differential neutrophil counts in all people who have recently had chemotherapy (p.166). (busulphan, melphalan, and procarbazine cause late myelosuppression (6–8 weeks after administration.)
- **Epidural or intrathecal lines for analgesia**: consider both meningitis and epidural abscess in people with long-term lines.
- **Lymphoedema, severe peripheral oedema, or peripheral skin damage including tinea.** Consider cellulitis which may present with very subtle changes initially.
- **Cough or shortness of breath**: community-acquired pneumonia or an infective exacerbation of long-term obstructive lung disease needs to be treated (p.264). A new pulmonary embolus may also present with fever, shortness of breath, and chest pain. Fever is likely when a pleural infarct has occurred (p.106).
- **Guarding or rebound tenderness on abdominal examination**: frequently encountered causes include diverticulitis, cholecystitis, and appendicitis.
- **Urinary frequency, urgency, or dysuria**: any of these symptoms requires further investigation. In unilateral complete ureteric obstruction, urine analysis may not demonstrate any abnormality (p.288).
- **Myalgias and arthralgias**: these symptoms suggest a systemic viral infection or the constitutional symptoms of any severe sepsis.
- **Stents**: biliary or ureteric stents can harbour infection which may be difficult to treat without changing the stent.
- **Vascular devices**: check cannulae or central lines including PICC lines. Always take a febrile set of blood cultures through central lines in a person who is and has these in place.
- **Known or suspected valvular heart disease**: continue to have a high index of suspicion for this being the primary source of sepsis or a 'sanctuary' site for the source of infection for recurrent sepsis (p.104).
- **Presence of ascites**: consider spontaneous bacterial peritonitis (or damaged bowel if there has been a recent drainage procedure) (p.144).
- **Recent or ongoing blood transfusion**: this may be a transfusion reaction. An incorrect cross-match is a medical emergency where the person develops fever and anaphylaxis.

- **Medications**: drug reactions may occur soon after commencing medications or months after ceasing a medication. This is often a diagnosis of exclusion.
- **Severe pain**: secondary to major insults such as bone fractures, a myocardial infarction, or gut ischaemia may precipitate fever.

Sub-acute onset (1–3 days) of fever
- **General influenza-like symptoms**: people with severe immunocompromise may develop symptoms and signs of sepsis over several days.
- **A palpable purpuric rash** suggests a systemic vasculitis (p.90).
- **Disseminated malignancy**: fever may represent progressive disease, new liver metastases, or a paraneoplastic phenomenon.

Acute-on-chronic fever
- **History of B symptoms**: the person with an established history of sweats, particularly at night, lethargy, and weight loss may mask underlying sepsis.
- **Previous treatment for sepsis**: the person may not have had adequate length of treatment or poor choice of antibiotics, and recrudescence of infection is likely in this setting. Areas of infection that may also have poor blood supply (such as head and neck cancers) may require longer courses of antibiotics. The other major cause for inadequate treatment is that there is an underlying fungal infection which has not been identified. CNS and respiratory tract infections are sites to consider. Any foreign substances (stents, valves, central venous catheters) need to be considered as sanctuary sites.
- **Endocrine disturbances**: hyperthyroidism may present with fever, tachycardia, and sweating. This may complicate a recent iodine load from radiological contrast (p.256).

Can you modify anything contributing to the symptom?

Life expectancy will be cut short by failiure to recognize neutropaenic sepsis. Urgently establish IV access, commence fluid resuscitation, and, having taken blood cultures (including from any central venous catheters), commence broad-spectrum antibiotics. Combinations include an aminoglycoside (with levels monitored every other day) and an anti-pseudomonal lactam (timentin or piperacillin) or ceftazidime.

Sepsis, even late in disease, should be treated if this will improve the person's comfort or function (including cognition).

In the late stages of a life-limiting illness, treating sepsis is rarely with the aim of changing prognosis but with the focus on achieving good symptom control. In the terminal phase (last hours or days of life before this infection), treatment would only be symptomatic.

Neoplastic fevers may respond to either dexamethasone 4 mg daily or NSAIDs (naproxen 750–1000 mg daily). Sometimes benefit will be gained from oral cimetidine 400 mg twice daily. Prior to commencing dexamethasone, it is important to exclude infection as the cause of fever.

Fevers from bone fractures, infarcts, or ischaemia may settle with management of the underlying problem. Regular paracetamol may be of benefit.

What underlying factors cannot be improved?

Recurrent or untreatable sepsis may occur in the setting of irreversible pathology. Infection distal to large airway obstruction or in obstructed urinary or biliary systems may be difficult to treat in the presence of continued obstruction. Systemic sepsis should be controlled, but recurrence is highly likely in these settings.

Symptomatic treatment

Non-pharmacological intervention

Fever should be actively treated with paracetamol (1 g four times daily orally or 500 mg four times daily rectally) in people in the terminal stages who cannot swallow and are febrile.

Pharmacological intervention

- Sepsis with an absolute neutrophil count of less than 1.0×10^9/l. (febrile neutropenia)
  - Cover: empirical broad coverage including *Pseudomonas aeruginosa*
  - Gentamicin 4–6 mg/kg daily IV plus ceftazidine 1 g every 8 hs IV or ticarcillin 3g/clavulinate 0.1 g every 6 hs IV.
  - Add vancomycin 1 g IV every 12 hs if person is severely shocked or known to be colonized with methicillin *resistant Staphylococcus aureus* (MRSA)
- CNS sepsis: intrathecal line
  - Cover must include staphylococci until Gram stain or cultures are available
  - Vancomycin 500 mg IV every 6 hs plus ceftriaxone 2 g IV every 12 hs
- CNS: epidural abscess
  - Cover for *S.aureus*
  - Flucloxacillin 2 g IV every 6 hs plus gentamicin 4–6 mg IV daily
- Lower urinary tract sepsis
  - Cover for *E. coli, Staphylococcus saprophyticus*
    — first choice: oral trimethoprim 300 mg daily 3/7
    — second choice: oral amoxicillin 500 mg + clavulinate 125 mg every 12 hs 5/7
  - Additional cover for *P. aeruginosa*: oral norfloxacin 400 mg every 12 hs 3/7
- Upper urinary tract infection
  - Ampicillin 1 g IV every 6 hs plus gentamicin 4–6 mg/kg IV daily in someone with normal renal function
  - In penicillin hypersensitivity, use aminoglycoside alone or ceftriaxone 1 g daily IV
- Lower respiratory tract sepsis
  - Cover for *Streptococcus pneumoniae, Mycoplasma pneumoniae, Chlamydophilia pneumoniae,* and *Legionella* species
    — first choice: benzylpenicillin 1.2 g IV every 6 hs plus oral roxithromycin 300 mg daily 7/7 (plus gentamicin if Gram-negative bacilli seen on sputum stain)
    — second choice: with a history of reaction to penicillin, ceftriaxone 1 g IV daily or, with
    — immediate hypersensitivity to penicillin, oral moxifloxacin 400 mg daily 7/7

- Empyema
  - Cover for *Streptococcus pneumoniae/milleri/anginosus*
    — first choice: ticarcillin 3 g + clavulinate 0.1 g IV every 6 hs
  - Cover for *S. aureus*
    — first choice: dicloxicillin 2 g IV every 6 hs
  - Cover for MRSA: vancomycin 1 g IV every 12 hs
- Cellulitis
  - Cover for *Streptococcus pyogenes* and *S. aureus* (especially with pre-existing wounds)
    — first choice: dicloxacillin 2 g IV every 6 hs
    — second choice (penicillin hypersensitivity): cephazolin 1 g IV every 8 hs
    — second choice (immediate penicillin hypersensitivity): clindamycin 450 mg IV every 8 hs
- Suspected infective endocarditis
  - Broad-spectrum cover until cultures available. Contact cardiothoracic surgery and infectious diseases as soon as possible
    — first choice: benzylpenicillin 1.8 g IV every 4 hs plus dicloxicillin 2 g IV every 4 hs plus gentamicin 4–6 mg/kg daily in normal renal function
    — second choice (history of sensitivity to penicillin): vancomycin 1 g IV every 12 hs plus gentamicin 4–6 mg/kg IV daily
- Biliary tree sepsis
  - Cover: usually Gram-negative sepsis
    — first choice: ampicillin 2 g IV every 6 hs plus gentamicin 4–6 mg/kg IV (plus metronidazole 500 mg IV every 12 hs if there has been previous biliary tract surgery)
    — second choice: ceftriaxone 1 g IV daily if previous hypersensitivity to penicillin
- Spontaneous bacterial peritonitis
  - Cover: Gram-negative bacilli *E. coli*
    — first choice: ceftriaxone 1–2 g IV daily

Further reading

Oxford Textbook of Medicine, Vol. 1, pp. 269–270, pp. 293–307.
Oxford Textbook of Palliative Medicine, pp. 284, 698.
Oxford Handbook of Palliative Care, pp.763–764.
Oxford Handbook of Oncology, p. 588.

Care in the last hours of life

Diagnosing dying

This is a diagnosis that clinicians must actively make.

The diagnosis of dying for most people with a life-limiting illness is an active diagnosis of an expected event. If there are unexpected changes in condition, clinicians need to exercise careful clinical judgement in the assessment of any easily reversible causes for the deterioration.

For most people with a life-limiting illness, the terminal phase of their illness is a progression of the systemic pathology—a final common pathway characterized by increasing fatigue and lethargy, anorexia, and weight loss.

This is a catabolic state in which there are few bodily reserves for unexpected insults such as infection. Once established, the cachexia syndrome cannot be reversed without addressing the cause of the life-limiting illness.

Progressive cachexia is seen in all life-limiting illnesses (cancer, end-stage organ failure, neurodegenerative diseases, or AIDS). Most obviously, this process is reflected in the rate of change of functional status—systemic change not related to the sites of symptoms or underlying pathology.

At first, the rate at which decline can be noted is measured over months, but this gradually accelerates so that the time period during which change can be recognized shortens. As this decline is noticed, ensure that long-term medications are reviewed and that the goal of each of these medications is known. Continuation of long-term medications should only be to prevent likely and immediate symptomatic problems as a person's condition starts to deteriorate.

The time period for change is also an estimate of future life expectancy. If function is declining by the week, prognosis is probably measured in weeks unless there is a clearly reversible cause for the deterioration.

The person who is dying from cachexia spends more time in bed, and is increasingly dependent on help with activities of daily living. The last hours or days of life are generally associated with:
- profound lethargy
- decreasing periods of wakefulness
- decreasing peripheral perfusion, often with progressive hypotension and hypoxaemia
- increasing clouding of consciousness or drowsiness.

What underlying factors can be improved?

Continue with symptom control medications at the doses that the person has required until this time.

The route of administration of medications may need to change as oral intake diminishes. Always use the simplest route of administration (e.g. sublingual) and avoid unnecessary use of infusion pumps. (people do not need to be attached to an infusion pump to have a comfortable death).

Symptomatic treatment

Non-pharmacological intervention

Ensure that the person is positioned for comfort. This includes avoiding putting someone with pleural effusion on the side with the unaffected lung in a dependent position or positioning the person to avoid painful areas (sacral pressure sores, known bony metastases).

Given increasing immobility, place the person on an air mattress whenever possible. This limits the number of times the person needs to be repositioned and helps with skin care in dependent areas.

Involvement of family/carers: if it is the dying person's wish, ensure that the people important in this person's life are aware that time is now measured in hours to days. Encourage people to continue to talk to the person and continue to hold and touch them, even if there appears to be little response.

Privacy: ensure an environment which balances privacy for the person and their family with excellent attention to detail in nursing care. Ensure that when the person is no longer able to ensure that they are adequately clothed or covered, caring health professionals attend to modesty.

Good mouth care: (keeping the mouth moist, especially if the person is mouth breathing) can involve both family and staff. This intervention is most likely to prevent the person from suffering a sensation of thirst.

Noisy respirations: if the secretions have pooled in the pharynx, provide the person with 30° head elevation. Reassure family and friends that noisy respirations in someone with a diminished level of consciousness are unlikely to cause distress to the dying person.

Breathlessness: check pulse oximetry and use oxygen if the person has an oxygen saturation that is less than 90 per cent. Ensure careful positioning to maximize respiratory function.

Acute confusional state: ensure a quiet and softly lit environment. Minimize noise from visitors. Ensure that visitors and staff provide quiet reassurance. Exclude urinary retention or constipation as a cause of agitation.

Fear or anxiety: this can be an overwhelming feeling at times for people at the end-of-life, even in the last hours of life if existential issues are at the forefront of their mind. Allow the person, if able, to describe their fears rather than provide false or glib reassurance.

Pharmacological interventions

Noisy respirations: ensure that this is not simply cardiac failure or iatrogenic fluid overload.

Use hyoscine butylbromide 20 mg SC every 4 hs regularly if there has been a response. Even with adequate treatment, noisy respiratory secretions can continue to be a problem. If cardiac failure/fluid overload is contributing to the problem, administer frusemide 20–40 mg SC immediately and apply a glyceryl trinitrate 25 mg patch. Reduce the fluid input.

With breathlessness, consider the use of regular opioids. In opioid-naive people, use morphine 2.5 mg every 4 hs regularly. In people already on opioids, increase the regular background dose by 30–50 per cent. Give a breakthrough loading dose of one-twelfth of the 24-hourly dose.

Acute confusional states: increase in frequency and severity as death approaches for many people. Treat with haloperidol 0.5–2.5 mg SC every 24 hs. In younger, less cachectic people (e. g. with primary CNS malignancies) higher doses may be needed. Alternatively, atypical agents such as olanzapine can be used, with wafers delivering medication to the buccal mucosa.

Fear or agitation: having excluded easily reversible causes and treated any delirium, consider a regular dose of a long-acting benzodiazepine such as oral lorazepam 1 mg every 12 hs or clonazepam 0.5 mg SL every 12 hs. Ensure that breakthrough SC midazolam is available (2.5–5.0 mg second to third hourly).

Crisis medications

There are times in palliative care when a catastrophic situation is encountered. This can include acute bleeding, choking, or suffocation. In such crises, it is important to ensure that the patient does not suffer. On such occasions in opioid- and benzodiazepine-naive people, one would use a crisis order such as morphine 10 mg IV together with midazolam 5 mg IV Absorption via the SC route may take too much time.

The issue becomes more complex when people are using opioids, benzodiazepines, or both. In such cases there would need to be at least a 50 per cent increase in the background dose of their medication .

It is imperative that these medications are made immediately available to ensure the comfort of the person and to acknowledge that the comfort of those around them—their family and friends—is equally important.

Further reading

Oxford Textbook of Medicine, Vol. 3, pp. 1405–1407.
Oxford Textbook of Palliative Medicine, pp. 1117–1134.
Oxford Handbook of Palliative Care, p. 735–748.

Section 2

Specific clinical presentations

Clinical pharmacology

Medications with a narrow therapeutic index

Many medications have a relatively narrow therapeutic index and, as such, need monitoring of plasma levels of free drug. Careful monitoring is needed to avoid toxicity and to ensure adequate therapeutic effect. These medications include:

- Antibiotics: gentamicin, amikacin, tobramycin, vancomycin
- Anticoagulants: warfarin
- Antiarrhythmics: digoxin, lidocaine, procainamide, quinidine, amiodarone, perhexiline
- Mood stabilizers: lithium
- Immunosuppressants: cyclosporin, tacrolimus
- Antiepileptics: carbamazepine, phenytoin, sodium valproate, phenobarbitone, primidone
- Other agents: theophylline, levothyroxine

Other agents with relatively narrow therapeutic indices for which routine direct plasma level testing is not available include oral hypoglycaemic agents, most cytotoxic chemotherapies, disopyramide, MOAIs (p.62), and insulin.

Further reading
Oxford Textbook of Palliative Medicine, p. 214.

Medications with non-linear pharmacokinetics

Most medications are eliminated by a *constant fraction* for each unit of time. The half-life in this model is constant at all times (first-order elimination). Elimination is exponential and a true half-life can be established.

When initiating therapy, a steady state will have been reached within five half-lives in this model. As medications are discontinued, within five half-lives there will be approximately 2 per cent of the medication left in the body (assuming a single-compartment model of drug distribution).

A small number of medications have non-first-order (zero-order) elimination where a *constant amount* of the medication is eliminated for each unit of time. This is seen when a substance is metabolized by a specific enzymatic pathway that becomes saturated. In this model, the rate of clearance fails to increase with increasing concentrations. Clearance is linear, and a true half-life cannot be established as the half-life increases as plasma concentration increases.

This means that a small increase in dose (e.g. 10 per cent) may lead to a very large increase in plasma level (e.g. 100 per cent). Conversely, drug clearance will appear to accelerate at lower levels.

In palliative practice, medications that have non-first-order pharmacokinetics include:
- phenytoin
- theophylline
- salicylates
- ethanol.

Further reading

Oxford Textbook of Medicine, Vol.1, p. 1010.
Oxford Textbook of Palliative Medicine, pp. 213–214.

Medications that interact with warfarin

Warfarin interferes with vitamin K-dependent clotting factors (factors II, VII, IX, and X), and with protein C and protein S production.

There are several ways that warfarin levels can be affected:
- modified drug metabolism (cytochrome P450 pathways CYP3A4, CYP2C, and CYP1A2) (p.72)
- those medications that displace warfarin from plasma albumin (p.70)
- changes in vitamin K metabolism, especially with changes to gut flora with antibiotic use
- hypothyroidism may reduce degradation of anticoagulation factors.

Any change in medication (or a substantial change in diet) warrants close monitoring of the anticoagulant activity of warfarin. There are multiple simultaneous pathways that unpredictably affect the level of anticoagulation.

Antibiotics likely to reduce vitamin K-producing gut flora sufficiently to increase the effect of warfarin are:
- broad-spectrum penicillins (piperacillin, ticarcillin)
- second- and third-generation cephalosporins
- clindamycin.

When choosing antibiotics, consider narrow-spectrum agents with less chance of changing gut flora: penicillin, amoxicillin, ampicillin, dicloxacillin, first-generation cephalosporins, and tetracycline.

Increased anticoagulation when on warfarin

Symptom control

Analgesics	Paracetamol, dextropropoxyphene
Antidepressants	SSRIs, venlafaxine

Anticancer

Hormone therapies	Tamoxifen

HIV/AIDS

Antivirals	Ritonavir

Intercurrent illnesses

Oral hypoglycaemic agents	Glibenclamide
Antiarrhythmics	Propanolol, amiodarone, quinidine
Antibiotics	Co-trimoxazole, erythromycin, clarithromycin, isoniazid, metronidazole, ciprofloxacin, tetracycline
Antifungals	Fluconazole, itraconazole, ketoconazole, miconazole
Antiepileptics	Phenytoin
Other agents	Alcohol (with liver disease), allopurinol, '…statins', methylphenidate, thyroxine, cimetidine, omeprazole, piroxicam

Decreased anticoagulation when on warfarin

Intercurrent illnesses

Antibiotics	Dicloxacillin
Antifungals	Griseofulvin
Antiepileptics	Phenobarbital, carbamazepine
Other agents	Vitamin K, sucralfate

Unpredictable effects on anticoagulation

Symptom control

Glucocorticoids	Prednisolone

Anticancer

Cytotoxic therapy	Cyclophosphamide

Intercurrent illnesses

Antiepileptics	Phenytoin
Other agents	Cholestyramine, ranitidine, '…statins', propylthiouracil

Medications that are contraindicated when on a monoamine oxidase inhibitor

There are two groups of MAOIs: irreversible inhibitors (phenylzine, tranylcypromine, isocarboxazid) which block type A (deaminates norepinephrine and serotonin) and type B (deaminates dopamine and tyramine), and reversible inhibitors (moclobamide) which reversibly block type A.

Non-reversible blockade of MAOIs can cause problems with:
- pethidine (hypertension, sweating)
- tramadol (serotonergic syndrome)
- dextromethorphan
- other opioids including morphine—use with caution (isolated case reports of hypotension, drowsiness)
- selegiline
- ephedrine (in cough/cold preparations—hypertension)
- amphetamines (hypertension)
- methylphenidate (hypertension)
- clomipramine
- venlafaxine
- SSRIs (serotonergic syndrome)
- oral hypoglycaemic agents (enhanced hypoglycaemic effects)
- insulin (enhanced hypoglycaemic effects)
- tricyclic antidepressants (serotonin syndrome)
- modafinil
- cheeses/aged meats/brewed beers

Further reading

Oxford Textbook of Medicine, Vol. 3, pp. 1320–1321.
Oxford Textbook of Palliative Medicine, p. 754.
Oxford Handbook of Palliative Care, p. 42.

Washout times for antidepressants

- Tricyclic antidepressants (amitriptyline, clomipramine, imipramine, nortriptyline, dothiepin, doxepin, trimipramine): taper dose by 25 per cent per day and then allow 2–4 days before commencing another antidepressant.
- SSRIs (citalopram, escitalopram, fluvoxamine, paroxetine, sertraline): taper gradually (25 per cent per day). Allow 2–4 days before commencing another antidepressant.
- Fluoxetine: allow 1 week before starting another antidepressant, except for MAOIs, when 5 weeks washout should be allowed.
- Venlafaxine: taper by 25 per cent per day and allow 1–2 days before starting a new antidepressant.
- Mirtazerin and mianserin: withdraw gradually (25 per cent per day) and then wait 2–4 days before starting a new antidepressant.
- Moclobamide: no withdrawal reported. Allow 1–2 days before starting a new antidepressant.
- Non-reversible MAOIs (phenylzine, tranylcypromine): gradually taper to minimize withdrawal side-effects. Observe a 1 week washout period when changing to another antidepressant except fluoxetine (5 weeks) or another MAOI (2 weeks). Continue a 3 week restriction on diet and other medications after discontinuation (p.62).

Symptoms associated with antidepressant withdrawal

With SSRIs, mirtazapine, mianserin, or venlafaxine, people may experience fatigue, myalgia, diarrhoea, nausea, light-headedness, dizziness, agitation, headache, or insomnia if long-term administration is stopped abruptly.

With tricyclic antidepressants, people may experience a syndrome of cholinergic rebound characterized by increased saliva, runny nose, diarrhoea, or abdominal cramping and insomnia.

Further reading

Oxford Textbook of Palliative Medicine, pp. 751–754.
National Prescribing Service Radar Number 35, *Targeting Depression in Primary Care*, August 2004.

Serotonergic syndrome

Serotonergic syndromes have been described with:

- tricyclic antidepressants and (any of) clonazepam, alprazolam (not available British National Formulary), lithium, SSRIs, thioridazine
- MAOIs and (any of) L-tryptophan, dextromethorphan, SSRIs, pethidine, or clonazepam
- single agent or combinations involving SSRIs, SNRIs, tramadol, sumatriptan, buspirone, carbamazepine.

Clinically, this syndrome may manifest with:

- changed mood (anxiety, agitation, restlessness, and hypomania)
- an acute confusional state
- neurological dysfunction including hyper-reflexia, increased tone, tremor and poor coordination
- autonomic dysfunction including tachycardia, labile blood pressure, tachypnoea, sweating, increased temperature, and sialorrhoea.

Serotonergic syndrome is a diagnosis of exclusion. Ensure that there are no infectious or metabolic causes for these symptoms and establish a temporal relationship with a seretonergic agent.

In a small number of people, there may be a marked rise in creatinine kinase.

A serotonergic syndrome is usually self-limiting and settles in less than 7 days. Stop the offending medication(s). Use anticonvulsants for seizures, benzodiazepines for any rigidity, and dantrolene for hyperthermia.

Raised temperature, raised creatinine kinase, and rhabdomyolysis leading to renal failure all carry a poor prognosis. Other complications with a poor prognosis include DIC (p.168) and seizures (p.210).

Palliative medications that require dose modification in renal failure

In most clinical settings, medications in established but stable renal impairment can be adjusted by either reducing the dose or increasing the dose interval in accordance with the degree of renal impairment. In the elderly, renal excretion of medications tends to decrease. (The volume of distribution also tends to increase in the elderly as muscle is replaced by increased adipose tissue.)

Renal elimination of a medication relies on glomerular filtration tubular excretion, or tubular resorption.

Medications that can worsen renal failure need to be stopped, if possible, if renal function is deteriorating.

Analgesics

Diamorphine, morphine, and codeine are all metabolized to morphine-3-glucuronide and morphine-6-glucuronide which are renally cleared. Dextropropoxyphene's metabolite norproxyphene can also accumulate in renal impairment, with reports of cardiac toxicity. (Fentanyl and buprenorphine do not require dose adjustment in renal impairment.)

Although glucuronide and sulphide metabolites of paracetamol are renally excreted, dose is not usually adjusted in renal failure.

NSAIDs cause a reversible fall in glomerular filtration rate in people with pre-existing renal impairment which may severely compromise renal function and cause hyperkalaemia. Indomethacin and diflunisal are renally excreted. Sulindac in equipotent doses may inhibit the cyclo-oxygenase pathway less than other NSAIDs.

Benzodiazepines

Diazepam metabolites can accumulate in severe renal impairment (GFR <10 ml/min). Nitrazepam, temazepam, and midazolam can be used.

Medications for frequently encountered comorbidities

Digoxin levels need to be carefully followed with changing renal function, with lower loading and maintenance doses. Amiodarone dose should be reduced for GFR <20 ml/min. Diuretics (especially potassium-sparing diuretics such as spironolactone, triamterene, and amiloride) and angiotensin-converting enzyme inhibitors should be reviewed carefully in people with worsening renal function at the end-of-life.

Antibiotics

Caution is needed with aminoglycosides and vancomycin in renal failure, with careful monitoring of trough levels on a regular basis.

For people with GFR <20 ml/min, adjust dose down by a percentage for the following: amoxicillin–clavulinic acid (50 per cent), benzyl penicillin (maximum of 20 mU/day), trimethoprim (50 per cent), piperacillin (50 per cent), and ceftazidine (75 per cent).

Anticoagulants

Fractionated heparin needs dose reduction in people with renal impairment. Monitor warfarin as it may be less protein bound. Hypoalbuminaemia leads to increased sensitivity to warfarin.

CNS medications

Lithium doses need to be carefully monitored.
Phenothiazines and butyrophenones do not need dose adjustment.
Reduce doses for vigabatrin and gabapentin.
Valproate and carbamazepine can be given unchanged.
Protein binding of phenytoin decreases in renal failure and more free drug may be found in plasma, requiring a dose reduction.

Oral hypoglycaemic agents

Gliclazide, glipizide, and gliquidone are the safest sulphonylureas to use but must be adjusted down if GFR <10 ml/min. Biguanides (e.g. metformin) should not be used if GFR <20 ml/min because of a prolonged half-life.

Bisphosphonates

Bisphosphonates can still be used in renal impairment, especially if hypercalcaemia is contributing to poor renal function. Use doses at the lower end of the range, and in people with significant renal impairment (<20 ml/min) infuse pamidronate at a maximum of 20 mg/h.

Further reading

Oxford Textbook of Medicine, Vol. 3, pp. 470–475.
Oxford Handbook of Palliative Care, pp. 42–43.

Palliative medications that require dose modification in hepatic failure

Hepatic function does not correlate well with changes in drug metabolism, plasma estimates, or potential toxicity.

Paracetamol (especially in the setting of chronic alcohol use, when glutathione stores may be depleted) may lead to unexpected toxicity.

Drugs bound to albumin may have a greater risk of toxicity due to decreased protein production (p.70).

In severe hepatic impairment, decreased first-pass metabolism may allow increased bioavailability, leading to toxicity.

When considering anticoagulants, not only can clearance of warfarin be reduced in liver disease but clotting factor production can also be reduced.

Medications which require dose reduction in severe hepatic impairment

Symptom control

Antidepressants	Amitriptyline, clomipramine (increased sedation)
Analgesic	Codeine*, morphine*, paracetamol[†]
Antiemetics	Metoclopramide
Benzodiazepines	Clonazepam*, diazepam*

Anticancer therapy

Antineoplastic agents	Cyclophosphamide, cytarabine, doxorubicin, methotrexate[†]; vinblastine, vincristine

HIV/AIDS

Antivirals	Indinavir, lopinavir, ritonavir (reduce in moderate hepatic impairment), saquinavir, zidovudine

Intercurrent illnesses

Antibiotics	Amoxicillin + clavulinic acid (increased risk of cholestasis), clindamycin, doxycycline, metronidazole
Anticoagulants	Warfarin, heparin[‡]
Antiepileptics	Carbamazepine[‡], phenobarbital, phenytoin
Immunosuppressants	Azathioprine, cyclosporin
Hypoglycaemics	Glibenclamide, metformin (withdraw)
Antihypertensives	Nifedipine, propanolol, verapamil
Antipsychotics	Chlorpromazine
Other agents	Allopurinol, theophylline, medroxyprogesterone, promethazine, ranitidine

* Avoid or titrate more carefully than usual in order to avoid precipitating encephalopathy or coma.
[†] Dose-related toxicity.
[‡] Reduce in severe hepatic dysfunction.

Medications that are highly protein bound

Medications that are highly protein bound will compete with other highly protein-bound medications. Displacement of a medication can lead to rapid rises in plasma concentrations because so little drug is normally free in the plasma.

Binding can occur to albumin, β-globulin, or α_1 acid glycoprotein. Renal failure, inflammation, fasting, and malnutrition will tend to displace medications from protein binding. (The proportion of a medication that is bound to protein can be considered to have no biological effect.)

Medications that are highly plasma bound and can displace each other include:
- warfarin
- aspirin
- phenytoin
- diazepam
- propanolol.

Medications that are metabolized by cytochrome P450

Cytochrome P450 is a family of haemoproteins responsible for metabolism, including many medications. Although predominantly found in the liver, they are also present in the wall of small intestines, kidneys, and lung.

Induction of enzyme pathways by drug A lowers the available levels of drug B (subtherapeutic levels) and may take as long as weeks to become clinically apparent. The same timeframe is required for effects to disappear once the relevant medications have been stopped.

Inhibition of P450 enzymatic pathways by drug A mean that more of drug B will be available (toxicity); this develops over days.

CYP3A4 accounts for the metabolism of more than 50 per cent of all medications. In order, the next most important pathways are CYP2D6 and CYP2C.

Further reading

Oxford Textbook of Palliative Medicine, pp. 216–217, 221–222.
Oxford Textbook of Medicine, Vol. 2, p. 1550.

Cytochrome P450 3A4 isoenzyme* (>50 per cent of all medications are metabolized through this pathway)

Substrates

Symptom control

Analgesics	Alfentanil, paracetamol, dextromethorphan, methadone
Antidepressants	Amitriptyline, imipramine, mirtazapine, sertraline, venlafaxine, fluvoxamine
Steroids	Cortisol, prednisolone
Antiepileptics	Carbamazepine
Benzodiazepines	Alprazolam†, clonazepam, diazepam, midazolam, triazolam
Other hypnotics	Zopiclone

Anticancer therapy

Antineoplastic agents	Cyclophosphamide, paclitaxel, vinblastine, etoposide, imatinib
Hormonal agents	Tamoxifen, testosterone, progesterone, flutamide, oestrogen

HIV/AIDS

Antivirals	Saquinivir, ritonavir, indinavir
Antifungals	Miconazole, ketoconazole, fluconazole, itraconazole

Intercurrent illnesses

Anticoagulants	Warfarin
Antibiotics	Clarithromycin, erythromycin
Antiarrhythmics	Amiodarone, digoxin, quinidine, lidocaine
Immunosuppressants	Cyclosporin, tacrolimus
Antipsychotics	Haloperidol, risperidone, ziprasidone, olanzapine, quetiapine, chlorpromazine
Antihypertensives	Amlodipine, diltiazem, verapamil, disopyramide, enalapril, felodipine, nifedipine
Other agents	'…statins', cisapride, omeprazole, terfenadine, loratidine

Inducers

CYP3A4	Carbamazepine, phenytoin, barbiturates, modafinil, oral contraceptives, cyclosporin, ritonavir, nevirapine, efavirenz
Antiepileptics	Carbamazepine, phenytoin, phenobarbital
Glucocorticoids	Dexamethasone, prednisolone
Other agents	Modafinil, cyclosporin, ritonavir, nevirapine, efavirenz

Inhibitors

Analgesics	Propoxyphene
Antidepressants	Fluoxetine, fluvoxamine, paroxetine, sertraline
Antibiotics	Clarithromycin, erythromycin, metronidazole, norfloxacin
Antifungals	Fluconazole, itraconazole, ketoconazole, miconazole, clotrimazole

Antiarrhythmics	Quinidine
Antihypertensives	Diltiazem, verapamil, nifedipine
Antiretrovirals	Indinavir, ritonavir, saquinavir
Antineoplastic agents	Imatinib
Other agents	Cimetidine, grapefruit juice

*This isoenzyme's activity decreases with age—lower doses will be needed for the same clinical effect (CYP2D6 function does not appear to change with age).

† Not available in the *British National Formulary*.

Cytochrome P450 2D6 isoenzyme*[†] (25 per cent of all medications are metabolized by this pathway)

Substrates

Symptom control

Analgesics	Codeine, oxycodone, morphine, methadone, hydrocodone, pethidine, tramadol, dextromethorphan
Antidepressants	Amitriptyline, nortryptyline, doxepin, desipramine, imipramine, citalopram, fluoxetine, fluvoxamine, paroxetine, venlafaxine
Antiemetics	Ondansetron

Anticancer therapy

Antineoplastic agents	Paclitaxel, vinblastine
Hormonal agents	Tamoxifen, testosterone

HIV/AIDS

Antivirals	Saquinivir, ritonavir, indinavir

Intercurrent illnesses

Antiarrythmics	Propanolol, metoprolol, labetalol, mexilitine, flecainide, quinidine, lidocaine
Immunosuppressants	Cyclosporin, tacrolimus
Antipsychotics	Chlorpromazine, haloperidol, trifluperidol, resperidone, olanzapine, cloazapine
Antihypertensives	Captopril
Other agents	Methylphenidate, dexamphetamine, omeprazole, loratidine, perhexiline

Inducers

Antiepileptics	Carbamazepine, phenytoin, phenobarbital
Antivirals	Ritonavir

Inhibitors

Analgesics	Methadone
Antidepressants	Citalopram, clomipramine, desipramine, fluoxetine, paroxetine, fluvoxamine, sertraline, moclobamide
Antiarrhythmics	Amiodarone, quinidine
Antipsychotics	Haloperidol, thioridazine
Other agents	Cimetidine

* This isoenzyme has genetic polymorphism.

[†] Two per cent of the population have multiple copies, leading to very rapid substrate metabolism.

Cytochrome P450 1A2 isoenzyme (>15 per cent of all medications are metabolized by this pathway)

Substrates

Symptom control

Analgesics	Paracetamol, methadone, phenacetin
Antidepressants	Amitriptyline, clomipramine, desipramine, fluvoxamine, imipramine, mirtazapine
Benzodiazepines	Diazepam
Antiemetics	Ondansetron

Anticancer therapy

Antineoplastic agents	Procarbazine
Hormonal agents	Tamoxifen, flutamide

HIV/AIDS

Antivirals	Ritonavir

Intercurrent illnesses

Anticoagulants	Warfarin
Antibiotics	Clarithromycin
Antipsychotics	Haloperidol, olanzapine, clozapine
Antiarrhythmics	Lignocaine
Antihypertensives	Verapamil
Other agents	Theophylline, caffeine

Inducers

Antiepileptics	Phenytoin, phenobarbital
Antivirals	Ritonavir
Acid suppressants	Omeprazole
Other agents	Cigarette smoke, cruciferous vegetables

Inhibitors

Antidepressants	Fluvoxamine, paroxetine
Antibiotics	Clarithromycin, erythromycin, ciprofloxacin, norfloxacin
Antifungals	Ketoconazole
Other agents	Grapefruit juice, cimetidine, omeprazole

Cytochrome P450 2C 9, 10, 19* isoenzymes

Substrates

Symptom control

Analgesics	NSAIDs
Antidepressants:	Tricyclic antidepressants, fluoxetine (CYP2C9), citalopram (CYP2C19), moclobamide (CYP2C19)
Antiepileptics	Sodium valproate, phenytoin, phenobarbital (CYP2C19)
Other agents	Tetrahydrocannabinol, diazepam (CYP2C19)

Anticancer therapy

Antineoplastic agents	Cyclophosphamide, paclitaxel
Hormonal agents	Tamoxifen, testosterone, progesterone

Intercurrent illnesses

Anticoagulants	Warfarin
Antiarrhythmics	Amiodarone, propanolol
PPIs	Omeprazole, lansoprazole
Other agents	Glibenclamide (CYP2C9), fluvastatin (CYP2C9)

Inducers (CYP2C9/10 only)

Antiepileptics	Carbamazepine (CYP2C19 also), phenobarbital
Glucocorticoids	Dexamethasone
Other agents	Ethanol

Inhibitors

Antidepressants:	Fluoxetine, fluvoxamine, sertraline (all CYP 2C9/19), paroxetine (CYP2C9)
Antibiotics	Clarithromycin, erythromycin, metronidazole, norfloxacin
Antifungals	Fluconazole, ketoconazole (CYP2C9/10)
Antiarrhythmics	Amiodarone (CYP2C9/19)
Antivirals	Ritonavir
Other agents	Cimetidine, omeprazole (CYP2C9/10), clopidogrel (CYP2C9), bupropion (CYP2C9), modafinil (CYP2C19)

* This isoenzyme has genetic polymorphism.

Cytochrome P450 2B6* isoenzymes

Substrates

Symptom control

Analgesics   Methadone

P450 enzymatic pathway inducers

Antiepileptics   Phenobarbital

* This isoenzyme has genetic polymorphism.

Dermatological problems

☼ Stevens–Johnson syndrome

- Severe blistering lesions of the skin, mouth, GIT, and conjunctiva.
- Initially, the skin lesions present as erythema multiformae on the palms and lips and then progress to other sites. Later, the skin lesions blister in the centre.

Causes of Stevens–Johnson syndrome

Frequently encountered causes	Less frequently encountered causes
Drugs	Viral infections
Sulphonamides	Neoplasia
Penicillin	
NSAIDs	
Anticonvulsants	
Sedatives	

History

Stevens–Johnson syndrome presents with a **febrile illness** associated with systemic symptoms of malaise, cough, myalgia, arthralgia, increasing shortness of breath (pneumonitis), rhinorrhoea, and conjunctivitis.

Skin lesions then develop. Typical **'target' lesions** have three rings: a bright red or pink inner ring, a lighter middle ring, and a dark outer ring. These will blister and desquamate.

In addition to the skin lesions, people may develop mouth or genital ulcers, GIT involvement leading to diarrhoea, and conjunctival ulceration.

Physical examination

- The presence of **skin lesions directs the diagnosis**.
- Examine the mouth and genitalia for ulcers.
- Examine the abdomen for right upper quadrant tenderness in the case of associated hepatitis.
- Evaluate the person's hydration status as there may be considerable fluid loss through the blistered lesions and diarrhoea. This is further complicated if the person has difficulty in swallowing due to lesions in the mouth and upper GIT.
- Ensure careful evaluation of the eyes.

Investigations and management

Prognosis measured in hours to days prior to the onset of this problem (symptom control)

- The major emphasis of care of these patients is supportive, regardless of their prognosis
- Despite the limited prognosis of this group, it is important to discontinue any medications that may be implicated.
- If patients have loose bowel actions consider octreotide (100 µg SC three times daily).

- Subcutaneous hydration may be appropriate if there are extensive blistering lesions or diarrhoea.
- Extensive skin or mucosal lesions may be painful, and adequate analgesia must be available. If skin damage is severe, use sterile paraffin for open areas.
- These patients may have conjunctivitis, and good eye care must be ensured.

Prognosis measured in weeks prior to the onset of this problem (in addition to symptom control)

- Check **FBC** for neutrophilia to suggest superimposed infection, and **serum electrolytes, urea, and creatinine** for renal function given large fluid losses.
- Check **hepatic function** as this syndrome may be complicated by hepatitis.
- If there are extensive blistering lesions and the person is febrile, consider superimposed infections of the skin and collect blood cultures.
- **Cease medications** that may be responsible.
- An urgent dermatological consult should be sought as biopsy will differentiate Stevens–Johnson syndrome from toxic epidermal necrolysis.
- Glucocorticoids do not change the resolution of Stevens–Johnson syndrome.

Prognosis measured in months to years prior to the onset of this problem (in addition to the above)

The mortality rate associated with this disorder is between 1 and 3 per cent. A poorer prognosis is associated with older age and more extensive skin lesion. Damage to the eyes may lead to permanent damage to sight, which in the worst case includes blindness.

Further reading

Oxford Textbook of Medicine, Vol. 3, pp. 828, 870.

☠ Toxic epidermal necrolysis

- Toxic epidermal necrolysis is a rare disorder that occurs mostly as the result of an idiosyncratic drug reaction.
- The development of skin lesions follows a flu-like prodromal illness.
- The skin lesions may quickly become very extensive and the extent of skin involvement dictates the prognosis.
- People with HIV and post-bone marrow transplantation are more likely to suffer this problem.

Causes of toxic epidermal necrolysis

Frequently encountered causes	Less frequently encountered causes
Antibiotics (sulphonamides)	Food additives
NSAIDs (oxicam)	Fumigants
Analgesics	Contact with chemicals
Anticonvulsants	
Allopurinol	

History

An influenza-like illness will precede the rash. This may resemble an upper respiratory tract infection with nausea, fatigue, and rhinitis. Later problems may occur, including conjunctivitis, pharyngitis, and pruritus.

Erythematous skin lesions then occur. These start on the face and chest and are often tender. The lesions then extend to the entire body and all mucosal membranes. The skin lesions are friable, and gentle pressure will cause the epidermis to slide off.

Physical examination

- Skin involvement is extensive. Depending upon the phase of the illness, there may be extensive sloughing of the epidermis, leaving a dark and oozing dermis. The nails may be involved.
- All the skin needs to be inspected including the perineal region. These people are likely to have extensive mouth, urological, respiratory, GIT, and genital tract ulceration. Examine for mouth ulcers, pleural effusion, and urinary retention.
- These people are at risk of **renal failure secondary to fluid loss**, and assessment of their fluid status is imperative.

Investigations and management

Prognosis measured in hours to days prior to the onset of this problem (symptom control)
- **No investigations are indicated**.
- Medications that are likely to be implicated must be discontinued.
- It is likely the onset of this problem will be a terminal event in this group and they must be kept as comfortable as possible.

- Subcutaneous or sublingual routes of administration will be ineffective. Intravenous access will be necessary to ensure that fluids, analgesics, and sedation can be administered.
- Insert an indwelling catheter. Ensure good mouth and eye care.
- Oxygen may improve comfort in people with hypoxaemia.

Prognosis measured in weeks prior to the onset of this problem (in addition to symptom control)

- The management of this group is supportive. This is not a group who would be considered for transfer to a high dependency unit. These people will require fluid replacement and reliable analgesia.
- **Dressings** of the desquamated areas should be done with sterile paraffin.
- If **diarrhoea** is present, treat with opioids or octreotide.
- These people are at risk of **bleeding**, and so crisis medications (p.52) need to be available.

Prognosis measured in months to years prior to the onset of this problem (in addition to the above)

This is a clinical diagnosis. A prompt dermatological consultation must be sought. These people require transfer to a high dependency unit for management similar to persons with extensive burns.

The following investigations and treatments must be initiated whilst transfer is organized.

- **Rehydrate** with 0.9 per cent NaCl IV.
- Check **serum electrolytes**, **urea, and creatinine** (pre-renal failure), **LFT** (hepatitis), amylase (pancreatitis), **arterial blood gases** (respiratory failure), **blood cultures**, **FBC**, and **coagulation studies** (coagulopathy).
- Commence **DVT prophylaxis** (enoxaparin 40 mg daily).
- Commence **PPI** (omeprazole 40 mg IV daily).
- Provide **analgesia** with PCA.

Mortality ranges from 10 to 70%, and is higher in older people with more extreme skin involvement. An early dermatological consultation should be sought to differenciate this from Stevens–Johnson Syndrome and to consider if IV intragram is appropriate.

Further reading

Oxford Textbook of Medicine, Vol. 3, pp. 870–871.

☠ Hypersensitivity reactions

- Systemic hypersensitivity reactions range from mild urticaria to major cardiovascular compromise (anaphylaxis).
- Urticaria without anaphylaxis is very common and may not require interventions.
- Anaphylaxis is a life-threatening medical emergency.
- This is an IgE-mediated event, which most commonly occurs within seconds of exposure to the aetiological agent. However, some responses may be delayed and the cause may not be identified.

Causes of anaphylaxis

Frequently encountered causes	Less frequently encountered causes
Radio-contrast	Medications (opioids, vaccines)
NSAIDs	Food (additives, fruits)
Antibiotics (penicillin, cephalosporins)	Idiopathic
	Exercise
ACE inhibitors	Blood products
Foods (seafood, nuts, eggs, cow's milk)	Cold/heat
Insect stings	
Inhaled allergens	

History

There may be rapid development of **urticaria** (raised pink papules and plaques all over the body) and **angio-oedema** (circumscribed swelling of the skin that causes a burning sensation). When these lesions occur in combination with **respiratory symptoms** (wheeze and shortness of breath), GI symptoms (nausea, vomiting, abdominal pain, diarrhoea), and **cardiovascular problems** (chest tightness, hypotension, tachycardia, and syncope), urgent assessment and management must be initiated. People may also complain of a **cough**, **widespread itching**, **headache**, **rhinitis**, and a sense of impending doom.

Physical examination

- Examine for **urticaria** and **angio-oedema**.
- There may be swelling of the eyelids, lips, face, and genitalia.
- Take the pulse and postural blood pressure.
- Auscultate the chest for **wheezing**.
- There may be widespread **abdominal tenderness** with guarding.

Investigations and management

Prognosis measured in hours to days prior to the onset of this problem (symptom control)

If there is a clear temporal relationship between the onset of the skin disturbance and the systemic symptoms the management is clear. Even at the very end-of-life, it may be appropriate to administer the following:

- adrenaline 1:1000 (0.3–0.5 ml) IM/SC
- dexamethasone 8 mg SC or hydrocortisone 100–300 mg IV
- cyclizine 12.5–25 mg SC
- salbutamol 0.5 mg SC.

This combination has been selected as these medications can all be given subcutaneously and are all readily available in palliative care units. The aim of these interventions is to alleviate wheeze and respiratory distress due to laryngeal oedema.

Simultaneously, abdominal pain should be managed with opioid analgesia and sedation provided for respiratory distress. Oxygen may improve comfort in hypoxaemia.

Prognosis measured in weeks prior to the onset of this problem (in addition to symptom control)

As noted above, if there is a clear relationship between ingestion or exposure to the development of the skin lesions and systemic symptoms, the management is not difficult.

Ensure IV access and start fluid hydration to maintain the blood pressure. Emergency management includes:

- adrenaline 1:1000 IM (0.3–0.5 ml) immediately and repeat in 5 min
- diphenhydramine IV 25–50 mg
- ranitidine 50 mg IV immediately and then three times daily
- hydrocortisone 100–300 mg IV immediately
- inhaled ventolin 2.5–5.0 mg four times daily if bronchospasm present.

It is important to keep these people under close observation as there may be a second phase of reaction 8–24 hs later.

Prognosis measured in months to years prior to the onset of this problem (in addition to the above)

If the diagnosis is not clear, these people require an ECG, cardiac enzymes, FBC, serum histamine, and tryptase levels.

Further reading

Oxford Textbook of Medicine, Vol. 2, pp. 1233–1237.
Oxford Handbook of Palliative Care, p. 804.

☼ Angio-oedema

- Angio-oedema is the clinical presentation of either a genetic or acquired deficiency of the C1 inhibitor.
- Angio-oedema describes the physical symptom of a circumscribed swelling of the skin, respiratory tract, or GIT.

Causes of angio-oedema	
Congenital angio-oedema	**Acquired angio-oedema**
HAE I	B-cell malignancies (multiple myeloma, Waldenstrom's macroglobulinaemia, B-cell lymphoma, chronic lymphocytic leukaemia)
HAE II	
Oestrogen-dependent angio-oedema	
	Medications (ACE inhibitors)

History

People present with recurrent episodes of **circumscribed swelling (angio-oedema)** but without urticaria. This is not itchy and is more likely to be described as burning rather than painful. This swelling may be found over any body surface.

Other problems include **GIT problems** (nausea, vomiting, diarrhoea, and abdominal pain) and respiratory problems (wheeze, shortness of breath, chest tightness).

Triggers to the attack include infections, medications (ACE inhibitors, oestrogen-containing medications), procedures, stress, and menstruation. A history of previous attacks or changes to medications must be sought.

Physical examination

- Attacks of **angio-oedema** may affect any part of the body, but often involve the extremities and the face. Typically the swelling is not red.
- The **abdomen may be tender** with guarding. People may be **dehydrated** due to fluid sequestered into the bowel.
- The voice may be hoarse, and there may be an audible wheeze. The presence of a hoarse voice indicates laryngeal oedema.
- Breathless and frightened people with an audible wheeze, using accessory muscles of respiration, are to be considered a medical emergency and immediate assistance must be sought.

Investigations and management

Prognosis measured in hours to days prior to the onset of this problem (symptom control)

People known to have hereditary angio-oedema who develop laryngeal oedema may still be more comfortable at this stage of life with administration of **C1 INH replacement** (500 U if <50 kg, 1000 U if 50–100 kg, and 1500 U if >100 kg) IV infusion. Despite administering the concentrate, crisis medications (p.52) must still be available in the case of acute respiratory distress as the onset to effect may be as long as 1 h.

If there is no laryngeal oedema, this group should receive analgesia and gentle fluid replacement.

People who present with angio-oedema *de novo* (in the absence of systemic symptoms or urticaria to suggest an allergic response) should not undergo further investigations. These people require analgesia, gentle fluids, and crisis medications (p.52) on hand with the onset of respiratory distress.

Prognosis measured in weeks prior to the onset of this problem (in addition to symptom control)

People who present with their first episode of angio-oedema should be investigated for **complement levels** (C4, C2). The aim of diagnosing hereditary angio-oedema in people at this late stage of life is so that, if necessary, they can receive C1 replacement with any subsequent episode. People with acquired angio-odema have antibodies to the C1 receptor, so they do not respond to replacement therapy. These people must have crisis medications (p.52) available as the risk of another acute episode of laryngeal oedema remains.

People with cutaneous swelling in the absence of laryngeal and gut mucosal involvement do not require intervention.

Prognosis measured in months to years prior to the onset of this problem (in addition to above)

Acute onset of angio-oedema with laryngeal oedema should be considered a **medical emergency**. These people require transfer to a high dependency unit for stabilization of their airway, fluid management, analgesia, and investigations.

In people with hereditary C1 deficiency, if C1 replacement is not available or the diagnosis has not yet been established, intubation and tracheotomy may have to be performed with severe respiratory compromise. Once these people have been stabilized investigations, should be initiated. This should also occur in people who present with milder episodes.

Additional investigations include:
- HIV, T-lymphotrophic viruses, and hepatitis serology
- LFT, LDH, EUC, FBC, and TFT.

An immunology consultation is recommended.

Further reading

Oxford Textbook of Medicine, Vol. 2, pp. 1233–1237.

☼ **Warfarin-induced skin necrosis**

- This is a rare but devastating complication of oral anticoagulant therapy.
- It has been linked to people with hypercoagulable states (protein C or protein S deficiency, factor V Leiden, antiphospholipid antibodies, cancer, people who have had heparin-induced thrombocytopaenia).

History

There is onset of numbness and tingling in well-circumscribed areas of the skin 3–7 days after commencing warfarin. Although this is the expected time of onset, the disorder has been noted in people years after commencing warfarin.

Following the sensory changes, erythematous skin lesions occur, which may be very painful. This is most likely to occur over the breasts, anterior thighs, and buttocks in women. Men have no particular pattern of skin involvement.

Physical examination

Initially, the physical examination may be unremarkable. Then, **erythematous lesions** surrounded by oedema may appear. These later develop into **haemorrhagic bullae**, which indicate full-skin-thickness injury. Later an eschar forms, resulting in deep scarring.

Investigations and management

Prognosis measured in hours to days prior to the onset of this problem (symptom control)

- Warfarin should be discontinued and vitamin K 10 mg IM/IV administered.
- Commence LMW heparin as the aim is to prevent a hypercoagulable state.
- Once bullae appear, the process is irreversible.
- Adequate analgesia must be administered.

Prognosis measured in weeks prior to the onset of this problem (in addition to symptom control)

- Adequate analgesia must be available.
- It is unlikely these people will be well enough for surgical debridement and so good wound care is essential.

Prognosis measured in months to years prior to the onset of this problem (in addition to the above)

It is likely these people will require surgical debridement and skin grafting of the deeper scars. An early dermatological consultation should be sought. Options for long-term anticoagulation should be discussed with a haematologist.

:✪: **Cutaneous vasculitis**

- Numerous vasculitic conditions present with cutaneous involvement.
- When the skin is involved, palpable purpura help make the clinical diagnosis.
- Cutaneous vasculitis should prompt consideration of systemic vasculitis, especially with symptoms of arthralgia, arthritis, haematuria, nausea, vomiting, diarrhoea, fatigue, or fever.

Causes of vasculitis
Infections: bacterial (especially streptococcal throat infections), viral, fungal, parasitic
Inflammatory disease: SLE, rheumatoid arthritis, Bechet's disease, inflammatory bowel disease
Drugs: penicillins, sulphonamides, allopurinol, amiodarone, streptokinase, thiazides, and warfarin
Paraneoplastic (especially breast cancer)
Idiopathic

History

People present with **purpura** although they may also have papules, vesicles, bullae, pustules, ulcers, or urticaria. These may all be painful, itchy, or both.

The associated **systemic symptoms** may include fevers, arthralgia, myalgias, haemoptysis, cough, wheezing, sinusitis, numbness and tingling of the extremities, abdominal pain, haematuria, testicular pain, weight loss, night sweats, and painful red eyes.

The onset may be **catastrophic** with an acute abdomen (bleed, rupture, ischaemia), acute shortness of breath (pleural effusion, pulmonary bleed, myocardial ischaemia), or anuria (acute renal failure).

Physical examination

- Examine the skin for **palpable purpura** and other skin lesions. Examine the mouth for ulcers.
- The eyes may be red and irritable (uveitis, conjunctivitis, retinitis).
- Palpate for tender sinuses.
- Inspect and palpate the hands and feet for joint deformities and digital infarcts.
- Auscultate the chest for a wheeze, fine crackles (fibrosis), or a pleural effusion. Check pulse oximetry.
- Examine for signs of heart failure (myocardial necrosis secondary to coronary artery inflammation).
- Examine the abdomen for tenderness and exclude an acute abdomen (pancreatitis, mesenteric angina or infarction, ruptured aneurysm, GI bleeding or gut oedema, intussusception).

Investigations and management

Prognosis measured in hours to days prior to the onset of this problem (symptom control)

This is a clinical diagnosis and further investigations are not indicated.

People who develop purpura without major systemic problems do not require intervention.

For people with systemic manifestations, it is likely that vasculitis will hasten death.

Prognosis measured in weeks prior to the onset of this problem (in addition to symptom control)

This group requires consideration of the precipitating factors. Interventions depend upon the severity to the episode.

- Mild cases may not require further treatments.
- More extensive cutaneous problems, without systemic symptoms require topical corticosteroids and antihistamines (promethazine 25 mg daily or twice daily).
- For severe cases, attention to symptoms and systemic corticosteroids is indicated (hydrocortisone 100 mg IV daily in a reducing dose).
- Treat hypertension if present.

Prognosis measured in months to years prior to the onset of this problem (in addition to prognosis measured in weeks)

This group requires investigations and treatment:

- **FBC, serum EUC, LFT**.
- **Urinalysis** spun for active sediment.
- **Immunological screen** (complement levels, antinuclear antibodies, ESR, CRP, rheumatoid factor, ANCA).
- **Skin biopsy**.
- **CXR** if there is clinical suspicion of infection or a pleural effusion
- If there is no response to corticosteroids, other immunosuppressive treatments may be necessary and immunology/dermatology consults must be sought as a matter of urgency.

Further reading

Oxford Textbook of Medicine, Vol. 3, pp. 388, 863.

Cardiovascular problems

☠ Superior vena cava obstruction

- In SVC obstruction, decreased venous return from the upper half of the body causes a rise in central venous pressure.
- The obstruction may be due to external compression, thrombus inside the vessel, or direct vessel invasion by malignancy.

Causes of SVC obstruction

	Frequently encountered causes	Less frequently encountered causes
Cancer	Lung cancer (especially small cell or squamous cell)	Lymphoma
		Mediastinal metastases
Intercurrent illness		History of mediastinal radiotherapy
		Recently placed central venous catheter (vessel trauma)
		Benign mediastinal tumours
		Thoracic aortic aneurysms
		Thyroid enlargement
		SVC thrombus

History

- With an insidious onset of SVC obstruction, people will complain of neck and facial swelling, headache or 'fullness' on bending or lying down, and increasing shortness of breath.
- In acute onset SVC obstruction, people often complain of dizziness and sudden onset of shortness of breath.
- Rarely, people may present obtunded due to cerebral oedema.

Physical examination

- On observation, **dilated veins** (neck, forehead, anterior chest wall) are often seen. Bloodshot conjunctiva may be present, with facial oedema.
- On occasion, there may be tachypnoea, proptosis, oedema of the arms and neck, and peripheral cyanosis. **Pemberton's sign** is elicited by putting their hands above their head and looking for facial flushing and hand veins that may not collapse.
- Assess airway patency as laryngeal oedema may cause life-threatening respiratory compromise.
- Assess cerebral function as cerebral oedema may be severe in the acute onset of an SVC obstruction.

Investigations and management

Prognosis measured in hours to days prior to the onset of this problem (symptom control)

- **Opioid analgesia** will be necessary for the relief of dyspnoea and headache.
- Check oxygen saturations and use **supplemental oxygen** if the person is breathless. The head of the bed should be elevated to 30°.

- **Dexamethasone** (16 mg/day) may reduce oedema.
- These people may be anxious and are at risk of seizures.
- In acute airway compromise, **crisis medications** (p.52) for sedation must be available.

Prognosis measured in weeks prior to the onset of this problem (in addition to 'prognosis measured in hours to days')

- **CXR** will be abnormal in 85 per cent of cases with a widened mediastinum and, at times, a right-sided pleural effusion. In the setting of gradual onset, there will be collateral venous circulation.
- **Chest CT** will demonstrate decreased or absent opacification of central venous structures and the probable cause of obstruction.
- Management of this group should include **a trial of dexamethasone**.
- If present, central venous catheters should be removed if possible.
- For extrinsic compression, **endovascular stenting** is the definitive treatment of choice. If thrombus is present, stenting can be combined with thrombolysis at the time of the procedure. Patency at 3 months is reported to be 78–100 per cent with recurrence rates of 7–21 per cent.
- **Anticoagulation** should be considered in the one-third of people who have thrombus associated with SVC obstruction. Anticoagulation should only be used if the thrombus is the *cause* of the obstruction and clinical evidence of obstruction is less than 5 days old.

Prognosis measured in months to years prior to the onset of this problem (in addition to the above)

- Once the person has been stabilized, **radiotherapy** may be of benefit in a number of cancers but symptoms can flare during treatment and the maximum benefit can take weeks.
- **Chemotherapy** should be considered in early SVC obstruction in tumours that are exquisitely chemosensitive (small cell lung cancer or lymphoma with an expected symptomatic response rate of 60 per cent). Median prognosis after the diagnosis of SVC obstruction is less than 3 months.

Further reading

Oxford Textbook of Palliative Medicine, pp. 248, 262, 598.

☠ Acute limb ischaemia

- Total limb ischaemia is a surgical emergency because without treatment the limb will be irrevocably compromised within 6 h. Amputation then becomes the only definitive treatment. People at the end-of-life are often unable to tolerate amputation.
- Limb ischaemia may be due to thrombosis, emboli, graft occlusion, or trauma.

Causes of acute limb ischaemia

	Frequently encountered causes	Less frequently encountered causes
Cancer		Pathological fracture (tibia)
		Extensive venous thrombosis
		Direct vascular invasion
End-stage organ failure	Stenotic arterial segment	Valvular heart disease
		Aortic dissection
	Atrial fibrillation with large arterial embolus	Cholesterol embolus
		Arterial cannulation (aortic balloon pump, angioplasty)
		Severe cardiac 'pump' failure with local thrombus formation
Intercurrent illnesses		Pneumococcal or meningococcal sepsis
		Intra-arterial drug administration
		Pelvic surgery (cystectomy or anterior resection where pelvic collaterals compensate for aorto-iliac disease)
		Thoracic outlet syndrome

History

- People often complain of the sudden onset of **severe pain** in the affected limb with altered sensation. Sometimes paralysis may occur. At times, the onset may mimic Raynaud's phenomenon.

Physical examination

- Early in the process, on observation, the affected limb (usually the leg) may have **blue digits**. When severe, the limb may be marble white, evolving over hours into a blue or purple mottled appearance as deoxygenated blood fills the skin. The skin will blanch on pressure. Darker mottling suggests local coagulation which will severely limit salvage of the limb. Fixed staining, blistering, or liquefaction indicate, a limb that cannot be salvaged.
- On palpation, the presence of peripheral pulses does not exclude significant vascular injury. However, absent pulse suggests complete limb ischaemia.
- An acutely swollen and painful limb raises the possibility of extensive venous thrombosis.

Investigations and managment

Prognosis measured in hours to days prior to the onset of this problem (symptom control)

This is a painful condition for most people. **Adequate parenteral analgesia is crucial**. If already on opioids, increase the dose by 25–50 per cent of their current dose. Remember that there may be a significant neuropathic component from nerve damage. In this situation, add ketamine (start with 100 mg SC infusion over 24 hs and titrate as tolerated) or clonazepam (start with 0.5 mg SC/SL twice daily). Consider spinal (epidural or intrathecal) analgesia early in people with complete and untreatable lower limb ischaemia.

Prognosis measured in weeks prior to the onset of this problem (in addition to 'prognosis measured in hours to days')

- These people require **urgent surgical consultation**.
- Ensure vascular access.
- **Check coagulation studies, FBC, and EUC**.
- Ensure **regular limb observations** are performed.
- **Doppler ultrasound** will demonstrate most accurately current arterial flow rates.
- The definitive study is angiography. However, this should only be performed in people who are well enough to tolerate any subsequent interventions.
- Incomplete limb ischaemia in the setting of a life-limiting illness can only be treated with anticoagulation and supportive measures. Complete ischaemia from an embolus needs urgent treatment if the person is well enough to tolerate it. This may include **surgical embolectomy**, **thrombolysis** (streptokinase or tissue plasminogen activator) and **fasciotomy** for compartment syndrome. If there is established ischaemia, consider **amputation**.
- In people who are too unwell to tolerate surgery, **percutaneous lumbar sympathectomy** (under CT guidance) may be useful. Following injection of the sympathetic plexus, some people achieve increased distal perfusion and a reduction in pain. However, the success rates are quoted as less than 50 per cent and some individuals may develop worse pain than that prior to the procedure.
- In the setting of severe venous thrombosis, **elevate, heparinize,** and **provide analgesia** (parenteral opioids). This is an extremely painful condition. In the group of people in whom no intervention is planned, consider spinal (epidural or intrathecal) analgesia early.

Prognosis measured in months to years prior to the onset of this problem (in addition to the above)

This is a **medical emergency**. A surgical consultation must be sought promptly. These people require angiography and either local thrombolysis or open embolectomy. Once surgically stable, anticoagulate and investigate the source of the embolus.

Mortality after embolectomy is 10–20 per cent because of the comorbid conditions that predispose to acute limb ischaemia and reperfusion injuries (compartment syndrome, muscle infarction, acidosis, hyperkalaemia, and myoglobinaemia).

Ischaemia secondary to trauma may require urgent surgical reconstruction.

People unsuitable for surgical intervention require consideration of sympathectomy. Combined discussions with surgical, anaesthetic, and radiology specialists are indicated.

⦂✪⦂ Cardiac tamponade

- In someone with unexplained dyspnoea or hypertension, consider cardiac tamponade.
- Its onset is often insidious with vague non-specific symptoms.
- The primary compromise is due to a rise in intra-pericardial pressure leading to decreased ventricular filling and decreased cardiac output.

Causes of pericardial effusion

	Frequently encountered causes	Less frequently encountered causes
Cancer	Malignant pericardial effusions	
End-stage organ failure	Uraemia	
Intercurrent illnesses	Acute viral pericarditis	People with pericarditis treated with anticoagulants for other reasons
		Following thoracic surgery

History

- People often describe dyspnoea and **tachypnoea** on exertion that progresses to air hunger at rest.
- **Postural symptoms** may predominate in people with hypotension.
- People may present **obtunded** or with a decreased level of consciousness.
- Other symptoms may include new-onset anorexia, dysphagia, or cough.

Physical examination

Physical findings need to be interpreted with care as findings are rarely 'classic'. A high index of suspicion is needed.

- On observation, neck veins may be distended, as may veins in the forehead, scalp, and ocular fundi.
- JVP may be elevated with a **positive Kussmaul's sign** (rise in JVP with inspiration). In rapidly developing tamponade, venous pulsations may simply be exaggerated because filling and filling time are both reduced.
- **Tachycardia** is frequent, although bradycardia may be seen, with uraemia or hypothyroidism as the underlying cause of tamponade.
- **Hypotension** with obvious shock and peripheral cyanosis are encountered late. **Pulsus paradoxus** (a drop of >10 mmHg of systolic pressure on inspiration) may be demonstrable. This will not be seen with severe compromise to cardiac output.
- An apex beat may still be palpable.
- Auscultation of the heart may reveal **muffled heart sounds** and a **pericardial rub**.

Investigations and management

Prognosis measured in hours to days prior to the onset of this problem (symptom control)

Investigations are not indicated. This is a clinical diagnosis. Treating dyspnoea with opioids and anxiolytics is crucial (p.24). The pre-syncopal feeling as blood pressure gradually falls can be very frightening for people, and sedation may be necessary.

Prognosis measured in weeks prior to the onset of this problem (in addition to prognosis measured in hours to days)

- **CXR** may show an enlarged globular heart.
- An **ECG** may disclose alternating polarity for any waves, most typically the QRS complex, and at times the P wave (electrical alternans).
- **Echocardiography** may disclose the volume of the effusion, the chambers of the heart whose filling is affected by increased pericardial pressures, and whether there is loculation of the effusion. An echocardiograph may also disclose the septa moving to the left on inspiration and to the right on expiration. Chamber collapse is likely first on the right side of the heart and subsequently the left. Low-pressure tamponade relates to right-sided changes, has few classic signs and occurs at pressures of 6–12 mmHg.
- Despite the limited prognosis of this group, a **pericardial drainage** should be considered.
- Ensure close monitoring while arranging a pericardiacentesis.
- Ensure that a large-bore cannula is in place.
- Check blood pressure frequently as circulatory collapse occurs without warning.
- Check **coagulation studies and platelet count** while arranging definitive treatment. **Discontinue anticoagulants**.
- In people with uraemic pericardial disease that is not causing critical haemodynamic compromise, intensification of dialysis may control the effusion.

Prognosis measured in months to years prior to the onset of this problem (in addition to the above)

In people with probable bleeding or clot in the pericardium, or in whom there is likely to be effusive constrictive pericarditis, a surgical approach is required through a subcostal incision to create a pericardial window, having drained the contents of the pericardial sac.

Further reading

Oxford Textbook of Palliative Medicine, pp. 262, 597.

⚠ Pericarditis

- Pericarditis is a local inflammatory response in both layers of the pericardium which may later lead to adhesions.
- Normal intra-pericardial pressure is negative but may became positive in the presence of inflammation, leading to impaired diastolic filling.

Causes of pericarditis

	Frequently encountered causes	**Less frequently encountered causes**
Cancer	Primary and secondary lung cancer	Mesothelioma
		Post-radiotherapy
End-stage organ failure	Renal failure	
Intercurrent illnesses	Idiopathic pericarditis	Bacterial (tuberculous pericarditis, pneumonia, rheumatic fever)
	Viral pericarditis (Coxsackie, Epstein-Barr, mumps, varicella, HIV)	Connective tissue diseases (rheumatoid arthritis, SLE)
	Myocardial infarction (acute, Dressler's syndrome)	Hypothyroidism
	Post-cardiothoracic surgery	

History

People most often present with **sharp localized chest pain** that worsens with respiration. Often, the most comfortable position for the person is sitting forward. Pain may radiate to the epigastrium, the left shoulder, or the trapezius ridge. Fever need not be present. Occasionally, dyspnoea or palpitations may be the prominent symptom. Non-specific symptoms may include hiccoughs or nausea and vomiting.

Physical examination

- A **friction rub** is often heard transiently in late expiration with the person sitting forward. The rub is described as a scratching or high-pitched grating.
- Evaluate for evidence of **cardiac tamponade**: cardiac decompensation including tachycardia, hypotension, elevated JVP, and muffled heart sounds (see p.100).

Investigations and management

Prognosis measured in hours to days prior to the onset of this problem (symptom control)

Parenterally-administered **antiinflammatory agents** (ketorolac 10 mg SC four times daily or dexamethasone 4–8 mg SC daily, or parecoxib 20–40 mg IV twice daily) are needed for adequate analgesia.

*Prognosis measured in weeks prior to the onset of this problem
(in addition to 'prognosis measured in hours to days')*

- An **ECG** shows widespread 'saddle-shaped' ST elevation with upright
  T waves early in the course of pericarditis, reflecting subpericardial
  inflammation. T waves may subsequently flatten and then invert over
  time. Over days to weeks, the ECG will normalize.
- **Echocardiography** demonstrates the volume of fluid and any cardiac
  compromise.
- **CXR** may show cardiomegaly. This only occurs in large effusions.
- **ESR** or **CRP** may be raised. Myocardial injury may be reflected with
  raised **creatine kinase-MB** or **troponin**.
- Other investigations include **FBC, EUC, TFT**, and **blood cultures** if
  febrile.
- If there is cardiac compromise secondary to a large effusion, symptoms
  may be improved by drainage.
- **Systemic NSAIDs** are the mainstay of treatment of uncomplicated
  pericarditis. In this group, treat with an oral anti-inflammatory
  (ibuprofen 400 mg three times daily with food). Ensure that this is
  given with meals and that either an H_2 blocker (ranitidine 300 mg twice
  daily) or a PPI (omeprazole 20 mg) is ordered. If symptoms
  continue, consider colchicine.
- Discuss with the cardiology service.

*Prognosis measured in months to years prior to the onset
of this problem (in addition to the above)*

- If a cause has not been found, other investigations should include viral
  serology, blood and fungal cultures, and auto-antibodies.
- People with renal-failure-induced pericarditis usually require **dialysis**.
- Ensure that **myocardial ischaemia** has been excluded as a cause of
  pericarditis.
- Between 15 and 30 per cent of people will suffer recurrent pericarditis
  especially in people with cancer or connective tissue disease.
- A small number of people will develop **cardiac tamponade**.
- **Constrictive pericarditis** may occur as a long-term complication. This
  may present as cardiac failure.
- If there is associated calcification, the treatment is pericardectomy.

☼ Infective endocarditis

- IE occurs when sterile vegetations within the heart become infected.
- If IE is untreated, mortality is high.
- There is high likelihood of sudden changes in condition, especially if heart valves or papillae are affected.
- In someone with known valve lesions, fever, and sudden cardiac decompensation, urgently evaluate for IE.

Causes of infective endocarditis	
	Frequently encountered causes
Cancer	Neutropaenic sepsis post-chemotherapy
End-stage organ failure	Any person with a pre-existing valvular lesion and sepsis.
	Post-dental work or poor dentition
	Post-procedure (urinary catheterization, cystoscopy)
	Respiratory, skin, gallbladder infections
	Unexplained recurrent sepsis

History

- **Fever** is common and tends to be higher with acute presentations and more pathogenic organisms. In the setting of life-limiting illnesses, fever may be totally absent.
- **Myalgia** is also frequently encountered.
- Presentations of chronic IE include anorexia, weight loss, fatigue, and night sweats—all symptoms commonly found in late-stage cachexia.
- **Embolic events** and **mycotic aneurysms** account for most complications in IE—CNS, splenic, renal, or hepatic compromise, or gut ischaemia.

Physical examination

A new cardiac murmur in the presence of fevers must raise the question of infective endocarditis.

Peripheral manifestations include petechiae (conjunctivae, palate, buccal mucosa), 'splinter' haemorrhages (sublingual lesions), retinal haemorrhages (Roth spots), nodules on digital pads (Osler's nodes) and nodular haemorrhages on palms and soles (Janeway lesions), clubbing, and signs of anaemia. Cardiac murmurs are almost always present except with early disease or tricuspid valve involvement.

Splenomegaly and petechiae represent long-standing disease. Embolic events most frequently cause neurological deficits but may result in abscess formation (brain, heart, kidney, spleen, GIT, and lungs).

Investigations and management

Prognosis measured in hours to days prior to the onset of this problem (symptom control)

Even late in life, treatment with **appropriate antimicrobials** is an important palliative intervention in order to avoid painful peripheral emboli or sudden new neurological deficits. The need for this is because the rate of embolic events rapidly diminishes after the initiation of appropriate antimicrobial therapy.

Prognosis measured in weeks prior to the onset of this problem (in addition to 'prognosis measured in hours to days')
- **Echocardiography** (including a trans-oesphageal approach in people with normal trans-thoracic studies) and blood cultures are needed for the diagnosis.
- **ECG** may show new atrioventricular, fascicular, or bundle branch block. In people with new ECG conduction defects, monitor until stable and exclude perivalvular abscess.
- Check **FBC** (with differential), **ESR** or **CRP**, **renal function,** and **urine analysis.**
- Continuing long-term anticoagulation in IE should be carefully weighed against the risk of haemorrhage at the site of emboli or mycotic aneurysms.

Prognosis measured in months to years prior to the onset of this problem (in addition to the above)
Consult cardiothoracic surgery early; there is decreased mortality in people who can tolerate surgery, with early surgery for perivalvular disease or ongoing sepsis despite appropriate therapy. If left untreated, IE has very high mortality rates, especially with virulent pathogens.

:☹: Venous thromboembolic disease

- VTED is often without symptoms or has non-specific symptoms for much of its clinical course.
- VTED is very poorly tolerated in people with other cardiorespiratory compromise.
- There is a need for a high index of suspicion as estimates suggest that 7–10 per cent of hospital deaths are related to PE, with 70–90 per cent of these people having no prior symptoms.
- The majority of fatal PE are identified at post mortem.

Causes of VTED	
	Frequently encountered causes
Cancer	Any cancer
	AML (M5)
	DIC
Intercurrent illnesses	Protein C deficiency
	Protein S deficiency
	Factor V Leiden
	Antithrombin III deficiency
	Antiphospholipid antibodies
	Recent surgery
	Prolonged bed-rest
	Recent CVA or AMI

History
People with a thrombosis arising in the deep veins of the legs (arms rarely and then mostly in the presence of a central venous catheter) may present with **swelling and pain of the affected limb**. Symptoms rarely occur until distally arising thrombus affects proximal veins.

Up to 50 per cent of people with an established DVT and no respiratory symptoms will have evidence of a PE on perfusion imaging.

People with PE may present with **acute onset of distressing breathlessness**. This may be associated with pleuritic chest pain. Ten per cent of symptomatic PE cause death within 1 h.

Physical examination
- **DVT** may cause pain, swelling, discoloration, and redness of the affected limb. Superficial venous dilatation may be seen. Diagnosis relies on a high index of suspicion.
- **PE** may cause tachycardia, tachypnoea, and hypotension. People may be cyanotic with increased respiratory effort (but its absence does not exclude PE).
- When increased respiratory effort occurs, individuals often appear very distressed and frightened.

- Findings of **right-sided heart strain** (elevated JVP, distended neck veins, loud pulmonary component of the second heart sound) or hypotension suggest serious haemodynamic compromise.
- **Pleural effusion and pleuritic rubs** are late manifestations of a pulmonary infarct associated with pleural inflammation.

Investigations and management

Prognosis measured in hours to days prior to the onset of this problem (symptom control)

Pain is a problem in many people with DVT. Compression stocking use should be delayed until collateral vessels have an opportunity to open up. Elevation will help to minimize pain. Arterial compromise due to massive DVT requires extreme leg elevation. Despite the short prognosis, anticoagulation with LMW heparin should be commenced (enoxaparin either 1 mg/kg twice daily or 1.5 mg/kg daily). Check the most recent renal function tests and calculate CrCl (Appendix 5). If CrCl <30ml/min, reduce the dose by half. This may help reduce swelling, improve pain, and prevent the development of a fatal PE.

Check whether or not this person has been previously anticoagulated and whether there were any complications.

People at the end-of-life who develop a PE may have **distressing breathlessness** and require prompt attention. Although investigations are not indicated, rapid symptom relief measures should be commenced. Commence opioids (p.24) and oxygen (aim to keep oxygen saturation >92 per cent to improve dyspnoea and chest pain by reducing pulmonary vascular resistance). Parenteral NSAIDs are useful for pleuritic pain. Sedation may be necessary if the person is distressed or frightened. Crisis medications (p.52) must be available.

Prognosis measured in weeks prior to the onset of this problem (in addition to 'prognosis measured in hours to days')

People in this group who present with a swollen painful leg are suitable for **venous Doppler imaging**. They should then be commenced on **LMW heparin** as above. Prior to commencing anticoagulation, **EUC, FBC**, and **coagulation studies** should be performed. As noted above, the aim of anticoagulation is to reduce the risk of fatal PE.

Acute onset of breathlessness in this group should be investigated with a **CXR, arterial blood gases** (especially in the presence of long-standing respiratory disease to guide oxygen supplementation), and the definitive examination of **CTPA**.

These people are best managed with LMW heparin (rather than warfarin).

Prognosis measured in months to years prior to the onset of this problem (in addition to the above)

If this is the first VTED episode, check levels of **protein C, protein S, antithrombin III, antiphospholipid antibodies, and factor V Leiden.** Also collect blood for **FBC, coagulation studies,** and **EUC** (calculate CrCl). This group requires aggressive interventions.

People with a high probability of PE without shock should undergo a **CTPA** plus an assessment of right ventricular function. If the ventricular function is not impaired, heparin (IV unfractionated heparin at 80 U/kg immediately, then infused at 18 U/kg/h to maintain the AAPT at 1.2–2.5 normal or LMW heparin; check with local haematology guidelines).

If there is shock or evidence of right ventricular dysfunction, thrombolysis should be considered. Failure to respond to thrombolysis in shocked people should lead to consideration of embolectomy.

Drainage of pleural effusions should only be considered if there are significant symptoms, given that anticoagulation must be suspended in order to perform drainage safely.

Haemodynamic compromise on presentation carries an acute mortality rate of 10 per cent.

Further reading

Oxford Textbook of Palliative Medicine, pp. 600, 909.

:☼: **Acute cardiac decompensation**

- Broadly, this is the clinical presentation of cardiac output failing to match tissue perfusion needs.
- Characterise acute cardiac decompensation as predominantly left- or right-sided.
- Most acute changes will be associated with left-sided systolic failure.
- Most people presenting with acute cardiac decompensation will have evidence of pre-existing (and known) pathology.

Causes of acute cardiac decompensation in people with known pump failure

	Frequently encountered causes	**Less frequently encountered causes**
Cancer	People with previous treatment with anthracyclines	Arrhythmias associated with direct myocardial irritation by tumour
Intercurrent illnesses	Recurrent episodes of acute myocardial infarction	Beriberi
	Anaemia	Viral cardiomyopathy
	Alcohol	
	Cardiac arrhythmias	
	Fluid overload	
	Poorly controlled diabetes	
	Mitral valve rupture	

History

- **Left-sided cardiac failure** is predominantly characterized by (in order) exertional dyspnoea, dyspnoea at rest, orthopnoea, and paroxysmal nocturnal dyspnoea (often associated with audible wheeze for the first time in this person's life).
- **Right-sided failure** is characterized by oedema, ascites, anorexia, and nausea.
- Remember that severe left-sided cardiac failure may present with right-sided signs.
- The presentation of **silent myocardial ischaemia**, especially in the elderly or diabetics, needs consideration when someone has unexplained cardiac compromise.
- In the palliative setting, **high-output failure** can be caused by anaemia or thyrotoxicosis, especially in people who have had an iodine load (IV radiological contrast or use of amiodarone) or sepsis.
- At the end-of-life, even **small parenteral fluid** loads administered for 'comfort' can precipitate acute cardiac decompensation.
- **Cerebral impairment** results from decreased perfusion and oxygenation.

- Distinguish acute cardiac decompensation from the clinical presentations of abnormal water and sodium retention or hypovolaemia causing shock.

Physical examination

- These people will look very unwell and tired. They may be breathless at rest or with minimal exertion.
- **Tachycardia** is frequently present with pulsus alternans (strong and weak pulses alternating).
- **Hypotension** may be the predominant finding in acute cardiac failure.
- **Decreased pulse pressure** and cyanosis highlight severe decompensation.
- On auscultation, third or fourth heart sounds may be heard.
- **Mid to late inspiratory crackles may be heard at the lung bases**, which may also be dull to percussion, consistent with pleural effusions.
- **Ascites, congestive hepatomegaly** (pulsatile in tricuspid regurgitation), and **dependent oedema** may be demonstrated. This may be worsened in the palliative setting because of hypoalbuminaemia.
- In chronic heart failure, **cachexia** may be the predominant finding.

Investigations and management

Prognosis measured in hours to days prior to the onset of this problem (symptom control)

People require rest, elevation of the head of the bed, and management of their symptoms. They do not require further investigations.

Morphine 2.5 mg IV/SC may be given as required for chest pain and breathlessness. Administer oral aspirin 100 mg immediately if they are able to swallow.

If there is chest pain, administer glyceryl trinitrate 600 µg SL immediately. Ongoing ischaemic chest pain should be addressed with regular opioids (morphine 2.5 mg SC every 4 hs if opioid naive, or increase the background dose and titrate to comfort) and topical nitrates (glyceryl trinitrate patch 25 mg daily). **It is possible to continue the management of cardiac failure when people are no longer able to swallow using:**

- furosemide 20–40 mg SC
- topical nitrates
- SC morphine
- oxygen may provide relief, particularly if they are hypoxic.

People who are peripherally shut down may require IV medications.

Prognosis measured in weeks prior to the onset of this problem in addition to 'prognosis measured in hours to days'

In this group, investigations directed to establish the cause of acute decompensation are indicated.

- IV access must be established
- ECG obtained to define cardiac rate, rhythm, and confirm an acute infarct
- CXR will demonstrate enlargement of the chambers concerned. Distended pulmonary veins with redistribution of blood to the apices will be seen in acute left-sided cardiac failure. Look on the lateral film for evidence of right ventricular enlargement in the retrosternal window defining fluid overload.

- Blood tests include **FBC** (anaemia, infection), **EUC** (renal failure, electrolyte abnormalities), **cardiac enzymes**, **TFT**, and **LFT** (congestive hepatic dysfunction).

The best management is to treat the cause.

- Anticoagulation (aspirin and LMW heparin) for acute myocardial infarction (exclude cerebral metastases, previous GIT bleeding, or recent surgery).
- Treat arrhythmias if they are causing the cardiac failure.
- Transfusion for anaemia.
- Carbimazole and beta-blockade for thyrotoxicosis.

Further management includes:

- **Rest, oxygen, and careful use of diuretics** (furosemide 40 mg daily or twice daily if not on diuretics or the addition of a second agent such as aldactone 50 mg twice daily if already on diuretics).
- **ACE inhibitors** (lisinopril 2.5–5.0 mg twice daily) or **angiotensin receptor blockade** (irbesartan 75 mg daily). Start with low doses as these people are likely to be frail and may be at higher risk of adverse effects.
- **Vasodilators, topical nitrates** (25–50 mg daily), or **oral nitrates** (isosorbide 30–60 mg daily) may decrease breathlessness by reducing the preload. Adverse effects of headache and postural hypotension will need to be monitored.
- **Digoxin** is of value in cardiac failure. In this group, it is probably not necessary to reach therapeutic levels rapidly with a loading regime. Ensure that renal function and electrolytes are normal and commence the person on an oral dose of 125 µg day. Repeat drug levels in 7–10 days. Monitor blood pressure, heart rate, and the onset of unexplained nausea carefully.

Prognosis measured in months to years prior to the onset of this problem (in addition to the above)

- **Echocardiography** is useful in determining chamber size, cardiac function throughout the cardiac cycle, and valve function.
- **Hypotension** (systolic BP<100 mmHg) indicates carcinogenic shock. This requires urgent transfer to a high dependency unit for inotrope support.
- **Hypertension** (systolic BP>180 mmHg) may indicate hypertensive cardiac failure. Examine for encephalopathy. Organize immediate transfer to a high dependency unit for IV labetalol. (Do not give SL nifedipine as this may cause an uncontrollable drop in blood pressure.)
- **Acute myocardial infarction** must prompt immediate referral to
- cardiology for consideration of thrombolysis or angioplasty with stenting.
- **Acute valve dysfunction** secondary to ischaemia must also prompt immediate referral for consideration of surgery.
- All other factors aside, presentation with cardiac failure and no reversible precipitant carries a median prognosis of only 6 months.

Further reading

Oxford Textbook of Palliative Medicine, p. 920.

☠: Cutaneous arterial bleed

- Arterial bleeding is a feared complication of many end-of-life illnesses.
- Although a sentinel bleed may occur, there needs to be a high index of suspicion for people with head and neck cancers, or extensive soft tissue involvement from sarcomas or melanomas.

Causes of major bleeding

	Frequently encountered causes	**Less frequently encountered causes**
Cancer	Erosion of the carotid artery in squamous cell carcinomas of the head and neck	Bleeds into any active tumour beds including cerebral tumours, cutaneous tumours, and sarcomas
	Intercurrent illness	
	Infection	
	Anticoagulation	
	Coagulopathy	

History

- **Head and neck cancers**.
- **Sentinel bleeds** can also occur from the mouth, nose, or ear. Severe local infection can increase the risk of bleeding.
- Any **cutaneous tumour**.
- Local trauma, recent antitumour therapy such as radiotherapy or chemotherapy (which may destroy a tumour that is stopping bleeding), or a coagulopathy all increase the risk of bleeding.

Physical examination

- Look for **local signs of sepsis** including erythema, swelling, and tenderness.
- For a potential cutaneous bleed, examine for local factors including evidence of compromise distal to the affected blood vessel.
- In head and neck cancer, palpate the carotid arteries and listen for bruits.
- Examine neurologically for any new evidence of ipsilateral Horner's syndrome, or lesions of cranial nerves IX or X.

Investigations and management

Prognosis measured in hours to days prior to the onset of this problem (symptom control)

It is highly likely that an acute bleed in this situation will be a terminal event. **Crisis medications** (p.52) for sedation must be readily available and may need to be administered intravenously. The aim is to ensure the person has no pain or memory of this episode if they survive. It will be crucial to deal with the fear that arterial bleeding engenders in everyone: the person bleeding, their family and friends, and clinical staff.

Red or dark green linen will help to reduce the visual impact of arterial bleeding. Apply gentle pressure to the bleeding site and ensure that the person is nursed in a single room.

Prognosis measured in weeks prior to the onset of this problem (in addition to 'prognosis measured in hours to days')

- If a sentinel bleed occurs, ensure that all **medications that may exacerbate bleeding are discontinued** (NSAIDs, heparin, warfarin).
- Check for a coagulopathy and correct if necessary (vitamin K 10 mg IV/oral, platelets, FFP).
- **Treat infection**.
- Commence oral tranexamic acid (500 mg four times daily) if there is no past history of VTED or haematuria.

If actively bleeding, decide whether this is a life-threatening situation. If it is life threatening, what should be done in the light of the known disease burden and overall condition? For example, in advanced head and neck cancer in someone with advanced cachexia in whom anticancer treatment is already exhausted, an eroded carotid artery is a terminal event and, for most, even the need for sedation is rapidly superseded by death. For a person with a smaller bleed, provide local pressure (with epinephrine-soaked gauze) and establish urgent venous access. Consider blood collection for cross-matching, FBC, and coagulation studies.

Prognosis measured in months to years prior to the onset of this problem (in addition to the above)

Once a sentinel bleed occurs there may be a role for radiotherapy or angiography and selective embolization. Even in this group catastrophic bleeding is almost certainly a terminal event.

Further reading

Oxford Textbook of Palliative Medicine, p. 636.

☠ Thoracic aortic dissection

- Thoracic dissections may involve one or more aortic segments (aortic root, ascending aorta, arch, or descending aorta). The most common site is the aortic root and ascending aorta.
- Ascending dissections are considered the most serious because of the possibility of impaired coronary and cerebral circulation, pericardial bleeding with subsequent tamponade, or acute aortic valve damage.

Causes of thoracic dissection

	Frequently encountered causes	**Less frequently encountered causes**
Intercurrent illnesses	Widespread atherosclerosis	Marfan's or Turner's syndrome
	Hypertension	Aortic arteritis
	Bicuspid aortic valves	Syphilis
	Chronic aortic dissection leading to aneurysm formation	
	Trauma	

History

These people may be asymptomatic prior to the presentation of a dissection (blood splits the aortic media) or rupture.

Most commonly, these people present with **severe chest and back pain**. The pain is often described as ripping or tearing. Pain that extends caudally suggests distal propagation of the dissection. Other symptoms may include limb pain or weakness (secondary to limb ischaemia or spinal cord ischaemia) and abdominal pain (mesenteric ischemia).

Occasionally, these people may present with any one or more of the following problems:

- increasing shortness of breath
- congestive cardiac failure
- acute myocardial ischaemia
- mass effect on large airways
- increasing dysphagia (pressure effect on the oesophagus)
- back pain and hoarse voice.

Physical examination

- These people will be **distressed and unwell**.
- They will be **hypertensive and display unequal arm pulse and blood pressure readings**.
- They may develop a new murmur of **aortic incompetence** (soft A2, high-pitched diastolic murmur occurring immediately after the second heart sound).
- Physical examination must include a full **neurological examination** (cerebral ischaemia, spinal artery ischaemia) and abdominal examination (mesenteric ischaemia).

Investigations and management

Prognosis measured in hours to days prior to the onset of this problem (symptom control)

This is a clinical diagnosis. No further investigations are indicated.

If the dissection involves the proximal aorta, this is likely to be a terminal event. People with distal dissections who survive the acute event still have a poor prognosis and remain at risk for subsequent dissections and rupture of a secondary aneurysm.

Regardless of the poor prognosis of these people, it is important to treat their **hypertension**. This will help prevent propagation of the dissection and rupture of the aorta. Initially the management should include labetalol 50 mg IV over 1 min, followed by a vasodilator (transdermal glyceryl trinitrate 25–50 mg daily). **The vasodilator must not be instituted first; if it is, reflex catecholamine secretion will occur, worsening the blood pressure control and increasing the risk of rupture.**

These people are likely to be distressed and anxious. **Pain** must be addressed with parenteral opioids and **agitation** with benzodiazepines (diazepam 5 mg IV immediately midazolam 2.5–5.0 mg SC immediately, followed by either clonazepam 0.5 mg SL/SC twice daily or midazolam 10 mg via SC infusion over 24 hs). Oxygen may help with breathlessness if they are hypoxic.

Prognosis measured in weeks prior to the onset of this problem (in addition to 'prognosis measured in hours to days')

This person is unlikely to be a surgical candidate, and further investigations are not warranted. The exception is when endovascular stenting procedures are available. Seek an urgent surgical consultation. If this procedure is available, further investigations and management will include:

- **insertion** of an **intravenous cannula**
- **blood pressure control (as above)**
- **ECG**
- check **FBC**, **EUC** and **coagulation** studies
- organize an **urgent chest/abdomen CT** or **MRI** scan to define the level of the dissection fully
- **analgesia**.

Prognosis measured in months to years prior to the onset of this problem (in addition to the above)

These people require simultaneous treatment and investigations, whilst organizing an urgent surgical consultation:

• **ensure intravenous access**
• **check EUC, FBC, cardiac enzymes, coagulation studies,** and **cross-match**
• **ECG**
• **CXR**
• **chest/abdomen CT or MRI**.

Surgical intervention must be considered in people with a proximal dissection except when they have suffered a neurological event. In this situation, the anticoagulation may cause an ischaemic event to haemorrhage, leading to severe neurological compromise. There is an estimated 30 per cent mortality for proximal dissections and 10 per cent mortality for distal dissections.

☠ Bleeding abdominal aortic aneurysm

- An untreatable symptomatic aortic aneurysm may be the reason for referral to a palliative care service.
- The 1 year mortality in untreated aortic aneurysms greater than 6 cm in diameter is 50 per cent.
- The risk of bleeding from an aortic aneurysm increases with its size: risk increases from a diameter of 4 cm, and increases rapidly from a diameter of 6 cm.

Causes of abdominal aortic aneurysms

	Frequently encountered causes	**Less frequently encountered causes**
Intercurrent illnesses	Widespread atherosclerosis	Connective tissue diseases (Marfan's syndrome, Ehlers–Danlos syndrome)
	Age	Chronic infection (tuberculosis)
	Hypertension	
	Hyperlipidaemia	Acute infections (brucellosis, salmonellosis)
	Smoking	

History

For most people, an **aneurysm is asymptomatic prior to rupture**. Pain is the presenting symptom of a ruptured aortic aneurysm. It typically occurs in the periumbilical region and radiates to the back, both the iliac fossa and the groin.

There are a number of patterns of rupture:

- Rupture into the peritoneal cavity. These people present with severe pain and shock, and then die.
- People have severe pain that has a biphasic nature, reflecting a small first bleed into the retroperitoneal region that is usually followed by a more substantial bleed. Following the larger bleed, these people appear critically unwell.
- Rupture into the duodenum (fistula between the aorta and the duodenum) will cause massive GI bleeding that is a terminal event.
- Rupture into the vena cava. These people present with pain, gross lower-limb oedema, and high-output cardiac failure.

Physical examination

- These people will be shocked and unwell.
- A pulsatile abdominal mass may be palpable.
- The abdomen may be **rigid, with guarding**.
- **Bowel sounds may not be audible**.
- Following a rupture into the caval system, a continuous loud murmur will be heard over the abdomen.

Investigations and management

Prognosis measured in hours to days prior to the onset of this problem (symptom control)

- These people must have **adequate analgesia**. If they are shocked, IV administration of medications is the most reliable route.
- Bleeding people are often **anxious**, and so benzodiazepines must be prescribed.
- A **very agitated person** will require benzodiazepines plus a major tranquilizer (chlorpromazine 25–50 mg IM if shocked or levomepromazine 25–50 mg SC).

Prognosis measured in weeks prior to the onset of this problem (in addition to 'prognosis measured in hours to days')

The main differential diagnosis is acute pancreatitis. Check serum lipase and amylase. It is unlikely that the person will recover from a ruptured aneurysm, but may stabilize from acute pancreatitis with hydration and analgesia.

Prognosis measured in months to years prior to the onset of this problem (in addition to the above)

This is a surgical emergency and immediate surgical advice must be sought. Immediate investigations and management include:

- plain abdominal X-ray (75 per cent of people with AAA will have calcification visible on plain X-ray)
- **abdominal ultrasound** will demonstrate the extent of most AAAs
- **CT or MRI** will delineate the extent of local bleeding
- ensure **adequate venous access**
- aim to **keep systolic BP at 100 mmHg**, initially with colloid and then blood as soon as this is available
- **urgent** cross-match, FBC, EUC, and coagulation studies
- **ECG**.

These people should be transferred to the operating suite as soon as possible.

The options currently available are operatively replacing the aneurysmal section of the aorta or placing a vascular stent. Both carry significant morbidity and potential mortality even in the setting of skilled clinicians.

Prognostic risk factors to predict mortality in ruptured aneurysms have been identified:

- age >75 years
- creatinine >190 µmol/l
- Hb <90
- loss of consciousness
- ECG changes consistent with ischaemia.

Three or more factors are associated with 100 per cent mortality from rupture. Two factors carry a mortality of 48 per cent and one factor carries a mortality of 28 per cent. Even if there are none of these risk factors, there is still a mortality risk of 18 per cent.

Gastrointestinal disorders

⚙ Oral mucositis

- Mucositis may be a complication of radiotherapy to the head and neck, chemotherapy, and bone marrow transplants.
- Mucositis may affect the mucosa of the GIT at any point, and is usually defined as oral or GIT mucositis.
- Oral mucositis may cause pain, decreased oral intake, and increased incidence of infections.
- Mucositis of the pharynx and oesophagus may cause dysphagia, odynophagia, ulceration, and perforation.
- Mucositis of the larynx may cause a hoarse voice, painful earache, cough, dyspnoea, and stridor.
- The WHO grades of oral mucositis are:
  - Grade 0: none
  - Grade 1: mild erythema, mild pain
  - Grade 2: oral erythema, mouth ulcers but a solid diet is tolerated
  - Grade 3: mouth ulcers; only a liquid diet is tolerated
  - Grade 4: oral alimentation is not possible.

Causes of oral mucositis

	Frequently encountered causes	Less frequently encountered causes
Cancer	Radiotherapy to the mouth, oropharynx, or oesophagus Chemotherapy for haematological malignancy aimed at severe bone marrow suppression	Chemotherapy containing 5-fluorouracil, cisplatin, or melphalan
Intercurrent illness		Apthous ulcers, widespread oral herpes simplex

History

- People with oral mucositis will complain of a **sore mouth**.
- The most important issue is to distinguish between inflammation due to therapy and other additional pathology such as **herpes simplex**.
- A history of previous cold sores in someone with widespread oral ulceration signals the need for **viral swabs**.

Physical examination

- Check **hydration status** (tissue turgor, pulse rate, blood pressure, and moisture of mucous membranes) and nutritional status if the mucositis has been severe (grade 3 or 4) or prolonged.
- Exclude other skin and oral lesions, specifically simplex lesions of the lips, oral candida, and evidence of more widespread mucosal/skin damage (Stevens–Johnson Syndrome (p.80) or toxic epidermal necrolysis (p.82)).
- If there is any question of a primary herpetic infection ensure that there are no central signs of encephalitis.

Investigations and management

Prognosis measured in hours to days prior to onset of this problem (symptom control)

In this group of people, further investigations are not indicated. However, these people all require **good mouth care**, with the frequency with which the care is attended seeming to be the most important issue. Agents that have been used include 0.9 per cent NaCl, sodium bicarbonate, and 0.2 per cent chlorhexidine. Care must be exercised if chlorhexidine is commenced as it can worsen pain because of the alcohol content.

Ensure that there are no colonies of oral candida.

People with oral muscositis, regardless of the severity, must have access to **analgesia**. This includes topical agents (benzdyamine) and systemic opioids. Best evidence exists to support morphine. In this poor prognosis group, morphine is most easily administered as SC injections. Whilst grade 1–2 oral mucositis may be managed with opioids as requested, people with grade 3 or 4 require regular morphine. The starting dose depends upon prior exposure and the overall condition of the person.

Prognosis measured in weeks prior to the onset of this problem (in addition to symptom control)

- Check FBC, EUC, and albumin.
- Hydration must be assessed and supplemental fluids administered parenterally (IV or SC) if necessary.
- Mouth care must be given as above.
- Pain management requires a combination of local and systemic interventions. Morphine is best administered by a PCA if patients are well enough.

Prognosis measured in months to years prior to the onset of this problem (in addition to 'prognosis measured in weeks')

Additional considerations include the management of superimposed infections and early consideration of **supplemental feeding** (TPN) while waiting for mucositis to settle.

Further reading

Oxford Textbook of Medicine, vol. 1, pp. 262–263; Vol. 2, pp. 533–534.
Oxford Textbook of Palliative Medicine, pp. 231, 241–242, 680.
Oxford Handbook of Palliative Care, pp. 126–127, 240–245.

:✪: Gastrointestinal mucositis

- GIT mucositis causes abdominal pain and diarrhoea. Other symptoms depend upon the level of the GI tract involved and include the following.
  - Upper GIT: anorexia, nausea, vomiting, melaena, haematemesis, ileus, perforation.
  - Lower GIT (including rectum): change in bowel habits, rectal blood or mucus, tenesmus, ileus, perforation, fistula formation.

Causes of GI mucositis

	Frequently encountered causes	Less frequently encountered causes
Cancer	Radiotherapy to abdomen or pelvis	Chemotherapy containing 5-fluorouracil, cisplatin, irinotecan, docetaxel
	Chemotherapy for haematological malignancy aimed at severe bone marrow suppression	

History

People will complain of **abdominal pain and altered bowel habits**. Other problems will depend upon the level of the GIT involved and may include nausea and vomiting, melaena, tenesmus, and the passage of mucus through the rectum.

Physical examination

- Check **hydration** and **nutritional status** (people can rapidly lose large amounts of fluid and protein).
- **Inspect** the **mouth and oropharynx**.
- Check **pulse, temperature, and blood pressure**.
- Palpate the abdomen for pain and exclude an acute abdomen.
- Ausculate for bowel sounds.

Investigations and management

Prognosis measured in hours to days prior to onset of this problem (symptom control)

In this group of people, further investigations are not indicated. Despite the poor prognosis, people who have diarrhoea or vomiting may benefit from parenteral fluids, either SC or IV.

Nausea and vomiting must be addressed regardless of prognosis. In the absence of an ileus or perforation, metoclopramide 10 mg SC three or four times daily may be used. Haloperidol 0.5–2.5 mg SC daily or cyclizine 12.5–25 mg SC four times daily may provide additional relief. In the event that this is a complication of chemotherapy or radiotherapy, consider the addition of a 5-HT$_3$ antiemetic (ondansetron 4 mg SL/SC/IV or tropisetron 5 mg SC/IV).

Pain and diarrhoea will require SC morphine. If diarrhoea fails to settle with regular opioids, SC octreotide (100 µg three times daily as a starting dose) can be used.

Prognosis measured in weeks prior to the onset of this problem (in addition to 'symptom control')
- Check **FBC, EUC** and **albumin.**
- Collect **stool cultures** for Clostridium difficile.
- If **pain** is a problem, parenteral opioids (morphine, hydromorphone) must be prescribed.
- People should receive either **ranitidine** (150 mg orally twice daily or 50 mg IV three times daily) or **omeprazole** (20 mg orally daily or 40 mg IV daily) for epigastric pain with the route of administration dependent upon associated nausea and vomiting.
- **Oral sulfasalazine** 500 mg twice daily may help with **diarrhoea.**
- In people with **rectal mucositis**, sucralfate enemas (20 ml of 10 per cent sucralfate solution twice daily) may provide relief from pain, tenesmus, and rectal bleeds.

Prognosis measured in months to years prior to the onset of this problem (in addition to 'prognosis measured in weeks')
- Consider endoscopy if symptoms persist for more than a week.
- In severe or prolonged cases, supplemental feeding (TPN) must be considered.

Further reading
Oxford Textbook of Medicine, Vol. 1, pp. 262–263.
Oxford Handbook of Palliative Care, pp. 126–127.

RTOG grading of gastrointestinal mucositis

Organ	Grade 0	Grade 1	Grade 2	Grade 3	Grade 4
Pharynx and oesophagus	No change	Moderate dysphagia or odynophagia	Moderate dysphagia requiring opioids	Severe pain and weight loss Parenteral feeding needed	Complete obstruction, ulceration, perforation
Larynx	No change	Mild hoarseness	Hoarse but able to speak, sore ear and throat, cough	Whispering voice, ear and throat pain requiring opioids	Dyspnoea, stridor, tracheotomy needed
Upper GIT	No change	Weight loss <5% from baseline Nausea and pain not requiring treatment	Weight loss <15% from baseline Opioids for pain	Anorexia with weight loss >15% from baseline Severe pain despite treatment	Ileus, obstruction, may require surgery Blood transfusions needed.
Lower GIT and pelvis	No change	Increasing frequency of bowel actions Pain not requiring treatment	Diarrhoea requiring medications Pain requiring opioids	Diarrhoea requiring parenteral support Must wear pads	Acute or subacute obstruction, pain, and tenesmus requiring surgery Blood transfusions needed

:⚙: Colitis

Colitis is commonly encountered in people who are unwell. It is often a major stressor on already compromised body systems at the end-of-life. Adequate assessment must include dealing with reversible causes late in the course of the underlying life-limiting illness.

Causes of colitis

	Frequently encountered causes	**Less frequently encountered causes**
Cancer	Radiation colitis	External pressure on two or more branches of mesenteric blood supply
End-stage organ failure		Hypotension
		Hypokalaemia
		Cardiac arrhythmia
		Atherosclerosis
		Pancreatitis
		Vasculitis
Intercurrent illnesses	Recent use of antibiotics	Medications (opioids, anti-cholinergics)
	Crohn's disease	
	Ulcerative colitis	

History

- *Clostridium difficile* accounts for about 20 per cent of all antibiotic-associated diarrhoea. Watery diarrhoea with abdominal pain, fever, and leukocytosis suggests pseudo-membranous colitis.
- **Diarrhoea may be bloody with colitis.**
- An **ileus** may develop late and be a prelude to toxic megacolon. This may mimic an acute abdomen.
- Check the degree of bleeding from the gut. Occasionally in Crohn's disease, bleeding can be local and high volume. Surgery needs to be considered.
- **Shoulder-tip pain and well-localized or diffuse abdominal pain associated with shock alerts to the possibility of gut perforation.**
- The severity of signs of colitis may be **masked by immunosuppressants or advanced disease.**

Ischaemic colitis occurs with
- vascular occlusion (thrombus, embolus, long-term radiation damage, and vasculitis)
- hypoperfusion (hypotension, hypovolaemia)
- vasoconstriction or venous compromise (pancreatitis, malignancy).

The gut may initially be hypermotile with poorly localized pain progressing to the intense abdominal pain of an acute abdomen (especially in uncontrolled atrial fibrillation).

In people with a known history of inflammatory bowel disease, be aware that withdrawal (or inability to take antiinflammatories or immunosuppressants), hypokalaemia, opioids, and other anti-cholinergics can precipitate toxic colitis.

Physical examination

Fever, dehydration, and tachycardia may be seen in all forms of colitis, including pseudo-membranous colitis. Specifically examine for atrial fibrillation and cardiac failure (ischaemic colitis). Examine for evidence of bruising or bleeding that may suggest coagulopathy. Include a full inspection of the skin for cutaneous vasculitis. The abdomen must be palpated to localize sites of pain which may give a clue to the underlying problem.

Abdominal examination may *not* have specific signs early in the course of ischaemic colitis, especially if there is not yet full-thickness gut wall compromise.

Investigations and management

Prognosis measured in hours to days prior to the onset of this problem (symptom control)

Regardless of the cause of colitis, pain and diarrhoea must be addressed. Analgesia is best given parenterally, preferably subcutaneously. Appropriate medications include morphine, hydromorphone, or oxycodone. These medications may also assist with management of diarrhoea.

In more serious cases, **octreotide** may be necessary. Other simple interventions to improve diarrhoea include discontinuation of prokinetic medications (metoclopramide, senna, domperidone).

Regardless of the stage of life, if *C. difficile* is considered to be the cause of the problem, causative antibiotics should be stopped and treatment with IV metronidazole or vancomycin commenced.

People with **ischaemic colitis** may be very unwell and this is likely to be a terminal event. In addition to opioid analgesia, these people may benefit from SC hyoscine butylbromide (20 mg four times daily) or octreotide to assist with cramping pain, and an anti-inflammatory agent (dexamethasone or ketorolac) if peritonitis has occurred.

Prognosis measured in weeks prior to the onset of this problem
(in addition to 'symptom control')

Check **FBC**, **EUC**, and a **stool specimen**.

A plain abdominal X-ray with colon diameter of >7cm suggests toxic megacolon. This is important to know, as there is a high risk of perforation. It is unlikely that these people would survive this, and crisis medications (p.52) must be available.

In the presence of clinical or biochemical evidence of **dehydration**, supplemental fluids may improve comfort.

The **management of diarrhoea** includes discontinuation of and prokinetic agents, and commencement of loperamide (two tablets immediately followed by two tablets after each loose bowel action) or atropine sulphate/diphenoxylate hydrochloride (two tablets three times daily). Octreotide (100 µg SC three times daily) is necessary in severe cases.

Definitively treat the diarrhoea of *C. difficile* with oral or parenteral metronidazole or oral vancomycin. Oral cholestyramine (1 g three times daily) may also be useful.

In **ischaemic colitis**, partial-thickness damage with no systemic manifestations of sepsis or haemodynamic compromise can be treated with gut rest and hydration. With full-thickness damage, surgery needs to be considered if comorbidities or prognosis will allow. The length of compromised bowel and comorbidities will dictate whether or not this is possible. People with inoperable ischaemic gut have a very poor prognosis.

Prognosis measured in months to years prior to the onset of this
problem (in addition to 'prognosis measured in weeks')

Investigations and management should be simultaneously initiated.

• **Blood cultures** if febrile.
• Ensure **IV access and commence hydration**.
• In the absence of perforation, further investigations include **abdominal CT**.
• Sigmoidoscopy will demonstrate raised 2–10 mm yellow plaques in the presence of pseudo-membranous colitis.
• If there is free air under the diaphragm, an **urgent surgical consultation** must be sought. Commence IV antibiotics.
• People with **ischaemic gut** should also have an **urgent surgical consultation**. If the damage is extensive or full thickness, excision of the gut section should be considered.
• Inflammatory bowel disease: where immunosuppressive therapy has been withdrawn, it should be reintroduced if possible.

Further reading

Oxford Textbook of Medicine, Vol. 2, pp. 493, 503, 613–620.
Oxford Textbook of Palliative Medicine, pp. 485, 492–493.
Oxford Handbook of Palliative Care, p. 260.

☠ **Upper gastrointestinal tract bleeding**

- A wide range of causes for upper GIT bleeding need to be considered in people with life-limiting illnesses.
- This is primarily a clinical diagnosis for which there needs to be a high index of suspicion. It may mimic other causes of systemic decompensation.
- Upper GIT bleeding is an emergency. Prompt investigation and treatment are crucial to minimize morbidity and premature mortality.
- About one third of GIT bleeds originate from the small bowel.

Causes of upper GIT bleeding

	Frequently encountered causes	**Less frequently encountered causes**
Cancer	Abnormal platelet function (cytotoxic agents, renal failure, NSAIDs, myelodysplasia, paraproteinaemias, acute myeloid leukaemia)	Gastric tumours Small bowel tumours
	Thrombocytopaenia (increased consumption, splenic pooling, decreased production)	
	Mucosal bleeding	
End-stage organ failure	Portal hypertension (oesophageal varices, splenomegaly, gastropathy)	
Intercurrent illnesses	Peptic ulceration	Mallory–Weiss tear
	Oesophagitis	Angiodysplasia
	Gastritis	Haemangiomas
	Sepsis (DIC)	

History

People often describe **nausea and vomiting** ('coffee-grounds' or haematemesis). **Melaena** may be reported but its absence does not exclude upper GIT bleeding. Postural symptoms may predominate in association with hypotension and hypovolaemia.

It is imperative to check if this person is currently or has previously received NSAIDs (including COX-2 inhibitors), corticosteroids, or anticoagulants. This increases even further with concomitant use of dexamethasone or prednisolone. Remember that many over-the-counter products contain NSAIDs, and must be specifically asked about.

Check a past history of alcohol use (in the long term), a history of chronic liver disease or previous GIT bleeding.

Physical examination

- Check conjunctiva and palmar creases for anaemia.
- Examine for **shock** (cold peripheries, a thready tachycardia, hypotension).
- Exclude an **acute abdomen** (suggesting perforation) and perform a digital rectal examination looking for melaena.
- Look for any evidence of **bruising or bleeding** to suggest a coagulopathy. A high index of suspicion is needed, as physical findings may be relatively normal in people even with significant bleeding.

Investigations and management

Prognosis measured in hours to days prior to the onset of this problem (symptom control)

Whatever the cause of bleeding, ensure adequate parenteral pain control. If the person is shocked, intravenous opioids may be more effective as subcutaneous absorption may be impaired.

Ongoing bleeding may cause **anxiety**. In this case, benzodiazepines (clonazepam 0.5–1.0 mg SL/SC twice daily, midazolam 2.5–5.0 mg as required or a starting dose of 10 mg SC over 24 hs) may provide relief.

GIT tract bleeding can cause **nausea and vomiting**, and regular antiemetics are indicated. It is usual to start treatment with metoclopramide (10 mg SC four times daily). The response to metoclopramide must be monitored. Alternative agents include haloperidol or cyclizine. Usually a combination of agents is required. Intractable cases may need chlorpromazine (25–50 mg SC) or levomepromazine (6.25 mg SC at night or via syringe driver).

Stop heparin, warfarin and review the need for NSAIDS or clopidogrel.

If **torrential bleeding** occurs as a life-threatening event crisis medications (p.52) must be available. Remember that torrential bleeding may be very distressing for the family or care-givers. In this situation, red or green sheets may reduce the visible evidence of bleeding.

Prognosis measured in weeks prior to the onset of this problem (in addition to 'symptom control')

- Define the likely cause of bleeding. It is very important to remember that catastrophic bleeding is unlikely to be reversible in this group.
- In this group, it is important to assess fluid status and hydrate if necessary.
- **Cross-match for a packed cell transfusion** at the same time as taking baseline bloods (Hb, renal function, coagulation studies, LFT).
- Low-flow **oxygen** may be useful if shocked.

- Correct a coagulopathy with vitamin K 10 mg orally or IV, FFP, and platelets.
- In the case of bleeding with an adequate platelet count, **tranexamic acid 500 mg** four times daily may stabilize blood clots. Use with caution with simultaneous urological bleeding as this may cause clot retention.
- If there is **upper GIT bleeding**, IV proton pump inhibitors (omeprazole 40 mg IV daily) or H$_2$ blockers (ranitidine 50 mg IV TDS) and oral sucralfate (1 g four times daily) may be useful.
- Octreotide may help reduce mesenteric blood flow.

It may be appropriate to consider **endoscopy** for localized injections, diathermy, fibrin, or banding of varices in this group. Surgery is rarely indicated in this patient population. If surgery would otherwise be the treatment of choice for uncontrolled bleeding but the person is not well enough, embolization through visceral angiography is an option in a selected subgroup.

Prognosis measured in months to years prior to the onset of this problem (in addition to 'prognosis measured in weeks')

This is a medical emergency. **Contact surgical teams urgently**.

- Examine the person for **shock**. If shocked, immediately insert two large-bore cannulae.
- **Cross-match** 6 U of packed cells.
- **Rapidly correct fluid loss** with colloids and packed cells immediately they are available.
- **Correct clotting abnormalities** with vitamin K, FFP, and platelets.
- If **bleeding varices** are suspected, commence octreotide 50 µg/h IV.
- All people should **receive IV omeprazole** (or locally available IV PPI).
- **Consider urgent endoscopy**.

If the person is not shocked, insert cannulae as above, collect bloods, correct clotting abnormalities, and transfuse if Hb <10 g/dl. A surgical opinion should be sought as soon as possible.

Further reading

Oxford Textbook of Medicine, Vol. 2, pp. 511–514.
Oxford Textbook of Palliative Medicine, p. 252.
Oxford Handbook of Palliative Care, pp. 276–277.

☹: Lower gastrointestinal tract bleeding

Approximately two-thirds of episodes of GIT bleeding originate from the lower tract.

Causes of lower GIT bleeding

	Frequently encountered causes	**Less frequently encountered causes**
Cancer	Malignancy (primary or secondary with direct invasion of the bowel wall)	
	GIT mucositis	
End-stage organ failure	Bleeding haemorrhoids (portal hypertension)	
Intercurrent illnesses	Diverticulosis	Inflammatory bowel disease
		Benign anorectal disease

History

- Rather than the altered blood of upper GIT bleeding, most people will describe **bright blood**. **Melaena** may still be present with bleeding of the terminal ileum.
- The larger the volume of bleeding in the proximal gut, the more likely that unchanged blood will be seen in stools.
- A history of previous episodes of lower GIT bleeding is important, as is any tendency to bleeding.
- Localized pain or tenderness suggests **diverticulitis** should be considered.

Physical examination

- Look for any evidence of a **coagulopathy** (peripheral bruising or bleeding).
- **Blood pressure drop** of >10 mmHg or a rise in pulse of >10 beats/min when standing from sitting suggests significant (>10 per cent) blood loss.
- Abdominal examination should seek any rebound, guarding, or tenderness to suggest an acute abdomen.

Investigations and management
Prognosis measured in hours to days prior to the onset of this problem (symptom control)

- Pain, anxiety, and nausea must be managed.
- Crisis interventions must be available. (p.52)
- Unnecessary medications must be discontinued. Stop any medications such as aspirin or anticoagulants that may worsen bleeding.

*Prognosis measured in weeks prior to the onset of this problem
(in addition to 'symptom control')*
- Examine for an **acute abdomen**. This may indicate **perforation**.
- A **plain X-ray** may show free gas under the diaphragm. This group is unlikely to tolerate major surgery, and this indicates that discussions with the family must be instituted and the focus of care changed only to comfort.
- Check FBC, EUC, and coagulation studies.
- **If Hb <10 g/dl**, a transfusion of packed cells may improve symptoms, especially breathlessness and anxiety.
- **Sigmoidoscopy** will assess anorectal sources of bleeding. **Colonoscopy** may be performed if the sigmoidoscopy is negative. Colonoscopy should not be performed if there is a concern about ischaemic gut or with suspected severe mucosal inflammation. Colonoscopy can definitively treat bleeding polyps, bleeding cancers, telangectasia, a nd arteriovenous malformations with either diathermy or laser. With no other known gut pathology, a labelled red cell scan or selective mesenteric angiography may localise bleeding and the latter allow selective embolisation to control bleeding.

*Prognosis measured in months to years prior to the onset of this problem
(in addition to 'prognosis measured in weeks')*
Consult the surgical team immediately.
- A large-bore cannula must be inserted and fluid resuscitation administered if shocked or haemodynamically unstable.
- Correct any bleeding diathesis with FFP and vitamin K.
- Discontinue medications likely to be contributing to bleeding.
- If febrile, culture and commence broad antibiotic cover.

Further reading

Oxford Textbook of Medicine, Vol. 2, pp. 512–514.
Oxford Textbook of Palliative Medicine, p. 252.
Oxford Handbook of Palliative Care, pp. 276–277.

☢ Bowel obstruction

- Small bowel obstructions due to late-stage malignancy are more common than large bowel obstruction.
- Twenty per cent of malignant bowel obstructions are multilevel.
- Up to 50 per cent of cases of obstruction in people with advanced cancer are due to causes other than the cancer.
- Rates of bowel perforation or strangulation complicating a malignant bowel obstruction are relatively low.

Causes of bowel obstruction

	Frequently encountered causes	**Less frequently encountered causes**
Cancer	Primary or metastatic cancers within the lumen of the gut, within the wall of the gut, or externally compressing the gut	Radiation strictures
		Infiltration of the myenteric plexus
		Severe constipation
	Primary or metastatic cancers of the peritoneum affecting gut motility	
Intercurrent illnesses	Adhesions	Intestinal hernias
	Inflammatory bowel disease	Sigmoid volvulus
		Constipation

History

- People with bowel obstruction most frequently present with an insidious onset of **cramping abdominal pain**, **distension**, and **nausea** and vomiting.
- In small bowel obstruction, **nausea** is an early symptom associated with copious vomiting, often of undigested food.
- Obstruction at any level can cause **faeculant vomiting** due to bacterial overgrowth with stasis.
- **Abdominal pain** is common, with both a constant dull ache and cramping pain being experienced. The pain is typically peri-umbilical for small bowel obstruction. Large bowel obstruction tends to be perceived more laterally. It may be initially less severe for large bowel obstructions. Incomplete bowel obstruction may present with severe cramping pain, followed by the passage of loose stools or flatus. In complete obstruction, the person passes no stools or flatus.

Physical examination

- Abdominal distension and visible peristalsis may be present but are not needed for the diagnosis.
- Localized or generalized abdominal tenderness may be present. Pain may be masked by corticosteroids or opioids.
- A palpable mass may be present.

- Bowel sounds may be hyperactive and high pitched, or absent.
  A gastric splash may be present in a high obstruction.
- Rectal examination may be unremarkable or reveal an empty and
  dilated rectum.

Investigations and management
Prognosis measured in hours to days prior to the onset of this problem (symptom control)
Investigations are not indicated.

Gentle physical examination should be undertaken to localize pain, and tenderness, and assess abdominal distension, and bowel sounds perform a rectal examination. If the rectum is full, a glycerin suppository followed by a Durolax suppository should be administered.

Analgesia with parenteral opioids must be available. In people with moderate to severe pain or evidence of an acute abdomen, these medications must be given around the clock rather than as required. This often requires co-prescription with antispasmodic agents when cramping pain and vomiting are present (hyoscine butylbromide 20 mg SC four times daily up to 120 mg via SC infusion, or octreotide 100 µg three times daily or via syringe driver).

Ranitidine (unlike proton pump inhibitors) will also reduce the volume of upper GIT secretions by 50 per cent. Ranitidine 50 mg SC can be given four times daily.

These people are usually **nauseous**. Vomiting is associated with more complete proximal obstruction and continued high input (both oral and parenteral).

The choice of antiemetic depends upon the clinical response and scenario. Although metoclopramide has prokinetic properties, it may still be considered the initial choice for control of nausea in this group. The individual will need close observation and monitoring to ascertain the effectiveness of the intervention. An increase in pain or vomiting should prompt a change in the regimen. Alternatives include haloperidol (0.5–3.0 mg SC daily) with cyclizine (12.5–25 mg SC twice to four times daily). Intractable cases may require ondansetron 10 mg wafers or via SC injection twice daily, or levomepromazine 6.25–12.0 mg via SC infusion.

Despite the fact that oral intake may exacerbate vomiting, people must be allowed whatever intake they find pleasing. Occasionally, very severe vomiting will be best managed with a NG tube to decompress a high obstruction. Each case must be assessed individually.

A mouth care regime must be instigated.

Prognosis measured in weeks prior to the onset of this problem (in addition to 'symptom control')
If this is the first presentation of a malignant bowel obstruction, the initial management includes the following:
- Gentle **hydration** with either IV or SC fluids.
- **NG tube placement** may be necessary to decompress the stomach, but most individuals do not require this.

- **Abdominal X-ray** (diagnostic of bowel obstruction with dilated loops of small bowel, more than three air–fluid levels, and no air in the rectum). Remember that in people with a functional obstruction, low tumour volume, or distal obstruction, plain X-rays may be normal.
- **Gastrograffin contrast studies** may be used to define partial obstructions or the site of a single obstruction.
- **Abdominal CT** scan may best define the cause of obstruction.
  The investigations will help indicate if any of the following interventions are considered to bypass, de-function, or alleviate the obstruction:
  - gastrojejunostomy
  - a laparoscopic de-functioning procedure (de-functioning colostomy, ileostomy)
  - percutaneous gastrostomy
  - expandable stent placement (gastric outlet, small and large bowel obstructions).

Surgical and stenting interventions are not indicated for people with multilevel obstructions. The challenge is to assess whether people are well enough to survive the catabolic pressures of surgery. If this is considered inappropriate, management should revert to that of people with a poor prognosis, with focus on symptom control.

Prognosis measured in months to years prior to the onset of this problem (in addition to the above)
The speed of onset of the problem and the site and completeness of the obstruction help to dictate the management.

All people will require the following investigations and management.

- **Abdominal CT scan**.
- Intravenous hydration and correction of electrolyte abnormalities.
- A grossly dilated large bowel, volvulus, perforation, or strangulated hernia requires **urgent surgical intervention**.
- Incomplete small bowel obstructions, multilevel obstructions, or large bowel obstructions secondary to constipation may be managed more conservatively. These people still benefit from a surgical consultation.

Further reading

Oxford Textbook of Medicine, Vol. 2, pp. 621–628, 780.
Oxford Textbook of Palliative Medicine, pp. 263, 496–504.
Oxford Handbook of Palliative Care, pp. 262–263.

① Ascites

- Ascites is defined as the pathological accumulation of fluid in the peritoneal cavity.
- The pathogenesis is poorly understood, and differs according to the underlying disease.

Causes of ascites

	Frequently encountered causes	**Less frequently encountered causes**
Malignancy	Secondary cancer (bowel, pancreas, breast, ovarian, lung cancer)	Hepatocellular carcinoma
End-stage organ failure	Cirrhosis (alcoholic, viral hepatitis, autoimmune)	Cardiac failure including constrictive pericarditis
Intercurrent illnesses	Pancreatitis	Protein-losing enteropathy
	Nephrotic syndrome	Malnutrition
		Budd–Chiari syndrome (hepatic vein thrombosis)
		Hypothyroidism

History

People describe **increasing abdominal girth**, at times associated with shortness of breath, early satiety, nausea and vomiting, and abdominal discomfort.

Fevers or an influenza-like illness raise the question of **spontaneous bacterial peritonitis**.

Previous episodes of ascites and risk factors for first presentations need to be explored. Associated portal hypertension with oesophageal varices (melaena, haematemesis) point to a hepatic cause. A sudden onset of ascites makes malignancy or Budd–Chiari syndrome more likely. In end-stage disease, ascites is often multifactorial.

Physical examination

Ascites is graded on its volume:
- **grade 1** (1–4l) is detectable only by ultrasound
- **grade 2** (4–8l) is detected clinically with evidence of shifting dullness
- **grade 3** (>8l) is associated with tense swelling and a fluid thrill).

Check for anaemia and jaundice. Look for stigmata of chronic liver disease including Dupytren's contractures, parotid enlargement, and spider naevi in the distribution of the superior vena cava. In males, gynaecomastia and testicular atrophy may be present. Check for hepatomegaly and splenomegaly. Always look for scrotal or labial oedema in the presence of ascites.

Investigations and management
Prognosis measured in hours to days prior to the onset of this problem (symptom control)

It is **not appropriate to investigate** the cause of ascites or to drain ascites in people who are this close to death.

It is very appropriate to ensure that the **discomfort and breathlessness** that are associated with gross ascites are managed with opioids. As previously described at this stage of life, the SC route of administration is the least invasive and most reliable. Ensure that the SC needle is not placed in an area that is oedematous.

Additionally, these people are often nauseated and may vomit because of a squashed stomach or hypomotile gut. It is often multi-factorial. Regardless of the stage of life, antiemetics must continue (metoclopramide 10 mg SC four times daily, haloperidol 0.5–3.0 mg SC daily, cyclizine 25–50 mg SC four times daily).

Prognosis measured in weeks prior to the onset of this problem (in addition to 'symptom control')

The only definitive treatment of ascites is to **control the underlying cause** of the problem. However, attention to **symptom control** is paramount. If there is tense ascites associated with respiratory compromise, pain, and nausea and vomiting, paracentesis is indicated.

Prior to an ascitic tap, it is important to establish whether or not a coagulopathy (platelets <40 10^9/l, INR>1.4) is present. There are no guidelines for the rate of fluid drainage. However, there have been reports suggesting that less rapid drainage may decrease the risk of a peritoneal bleed.

Whilst 90 per cent of people will receive relief of symptoms when ascites is drained, there may be **adverse effects**. These include hypovolaemia and hypotension, renal dysfunction (less likely if there is peripheral oedema), perforated viscus, peritonitis, and fistula formation.

In the management of non-malignant ascites, guidelines support the benefit of concentrated albumin replacement when more than 5l of fluid is drained (replace 8 g/l of fluid drained). Regardless of the volumes to be drained, if the person is taking diuretics, these must be stopped for the 24h each side of the tap.

Prognosis measured in months to years prior to the onset of this problem (in addition to the above)

- Establish a cause for ascites.
- **FBC** looking for anaemia or neutrophilia. Check coagulation studies.
- **Ultrasound** will define hepatic metastases or cirrhosis.
- **Doppler studies** will assess patency of the hepatic and portal veins.
- **Abdominal paracentesis** and **analysis of peritoneal fluid** will help establish a primary cause. Fluid should be analysed for cell count (<250/dl is normal), microscopy, cytology, protein and albumin, amylase, and culture.
- Check serum protein and albumin, liver and renal function, and serum amylase.

- Serum to ascites albumin gradient (SAAG) can help in the differential cause (>11 g/l probably due to cirrhosis, fulminant hepatic, failure, liver metastases, alcoholic hepatitis, or cardiac failure).
- Turbid ascites is seen in pancreatitis or tuberculosis.
- White (chylous) fluid suggests lymphatic obstruction.
- People with malignant ascites should receive an oncology consultation for consideration of any chemotherapeutic options.

In non-malignant ascites, **diuretics** are the initial choice for symptomatic management of ascites. The first diuretic of choice is spironolactone (100 mg twice daily) and a loop diuretic (furosemide 40–80 mg daily) if tolerated. With adequate doses, a response may be seen in a few days, but postural symptoms, renal impairment and electrolyte abnormalities may limit the efficacy of the intervention. This approach is often utilized for the management of malignant ascites, but with less evidence to support the practice.

When considering the management of **malignant ascites**, the need for repeated paracentesis may be more effectively managed with permanent peritoneal drain placement.

In people with a shorter prognosis months, **placement of a tunnel catheter** (Tenckoff catheter or modified venous port) with an external portal for drainage may be effective.

In people with a longer prognosis (years), **a peritoneal–venous** shunt may be useful. There are complications associated with this procedure, especially DIC. It has been suggested that completely draining the ascites prior to the procedure can help limit this complication.

Other treatment strategies under investigation include the use of octreotide, intraperitoneal chemotherapy, and radioisotopes. There is no role for salt and water restriction or bed-rest in malignant ascites.

Ascites associated with cirrhosis carries a poor prognosis, with median survival of 2 years. Except for ovarian and breast cancer, the development of malignant ascites carries a median prognosis of 3 months.

Further reading

Oxford Textbook of Medicine, Vol. 2, pp. 733–741.
Oxford Textbook of Palliative Medicine, pp. 507, 512–515.
Oxford Handbook of Palliative Care, pp. 268–270.

☼ Biliary sepsis

- Acute cholangitis is a life-threatening complication of biliary obstruction.
- Cholangitis occurs when the normally sterile bile is affected by ascending infections.
- This is most commonly due to translocation of bacteria from the portal system or introduced by biliary instrumentation.
- Early diagnosis is necessary to minimize the high mortality rate associated with biliary sepsis, especially in the elderly or people with significant comorbidities.

Causes of biliary sepsis

	Frequently encountered causes	Less frequently encountered causes
Cancer	Carcinoma of the pancreas	Duodenal carcinoma
	Cholangiocarcinoma or disease around the porta hepatis	
End-stage organ failure		Post-liver transplant
Intercurrent illnesses	Biliary stones (choledocholithiasis, hepatolithiasis)	Primary sclerosing cholangitis
	Pancreatitis	Biliary surgery
	Post-ERCP	AIDS (benign stricture)
	Change of biliary stent	Spontaneous or surgical biliary–enteric fistula

History

The classical presentation of **fevers, jaundice, and right upper quadrant pain (Charcot's triad)** is usually a late presentation. If this is associated with drowsiness, confusion, and shock, the **prognosis is poor**.

Most people present with more non-specific signs of **fluctuating fever, nausea and vomiting, and abdominal pain** (which may be generalized). Sometimes **pain** may mimic angina or radiate to the right shoulder tip.

When obstruction is present, expect individuals to describe dark urine and pale stools.

Physical examination

- In acute cholangitis, severe pain on inspiration while palpating the right upper quadrant (**Murphy's sign**) may be positive.
- Additional physical findings include **fever, jaundice, abdominal distension, and signs of peritonism**.
- In malignant obstruction of biliary flow, a painless palpable gall bladder (**Courvoisier's sign**) may be positive.

Investigations and management

Prognosis measured in hours to days prior to the onset of this problem (symptom control)

- Acute cholangitis is a life-threatening condition with a high mortality.
- Worse prognostic features include old age and acute renal failure.
- In the very final stages of life, it may not be appropriate to commence regular antibiotics.
- Possible symptoms include pain. At this stage, pain is best managed with SC opioids.
- People may have pruritus, and if these people have pain, the opioid of choice is hydromorphone which may cause less itching than other opioids.
- Other symptoms include nausea and vomiting and fever. The management of fever is both pharmacological (regular paracetamol 1 g four times daily, oral/IV/rectal 500 mg four times daily, and non-pharmacological (tepid sponge, fan, and cool ambient temperatures).
- People with jaundice may develop itch. The **itch of cholestasis** may be relieved by relieving the obstruction, but symptomatic treatments include 5-HT$_3$ antagonists as first-line therapy or an androgen (methyltestosterone 25 mg SL). Non-pharmacological measures to address itch include avoiding and treating anxiety and treating insomnia. Ensure that the skin is not dry and discourage the use of soap. Ensure that the person's room is not overheated. Maintain hydration.

Prognosis measured in weeks prior to the onset of this problem (in addition to 'symptom control')

These people may be **shocked**. **Fluid resuscitation**, **pain relief**, **antiemetics and broad-spectrum antibiotics** should be initiated (IV ampicillin 2g every 6h and gentamicin 4–6mg/kg IV daily). Prior to commencing antibiotics, blood should be drawn for blood cultures. Further investigations should include **FBC, LFTs, and coagulation studies**.

LFTs are usually abnormal, with a cholestatic picture (raised GGT, alkaline phosphatase, and bilirubin). Transaminases may also be elevated and suggest a hepatic cause rather than biliary pathology. In elderly or debilitated people, WCC may be normal, reflecting an inability to mount an inflammatory response.

If **INR>1.4**, commence vitamin K 10 mg IV or orally daily.

A **biliary ultrasound** may identify the cause of the obstruction.

In someone with no obvious cause, an ERCP may be considered.

Despite the poor prognosis of these people, **endoscopic** or **percutaneous drainage** of a dilated biliary tree may provide good symptom relief.

Prognosis measured in months to years prior to the onset of this problem (in addition to the above)

Once stabilized, **laparoscopic or open cholecystectomy** should be performed.

Further reading

Oxford Textbook of Medicine, Vol. 2, pp. 700–713.
Oxford Handbook of Palliative Care, p. 292.

☼ Acute pancreatitis

- Pancreatitis occurs after an inflammatory reaction is triggered within the pancreas.
- It is divided into mild acute pancreatitis, severe acute pancreatitis, and chronic pancreatitis.
- The classification of severe pancreatitis is made when any of the following is present:
  1. Organ failure with one or more of the following:
     - shock (systolic blood pressure <90 mmHg)
     - pulmonary insufficiency (PaO_2 ≤60 mmHg)
     - renal failure (serum creatinine level >180 µmol/l after rehydration)
     - GIT bleeding (>500 ml in 24 hs).
  2. Local complications such as necrosis, pseudocyst, or abscess.
  3. At least three of Ranson's criteria:
     - age >55 years
     - WCC >16×10^9/litre
     - blood glucose >11 mmol/l
     - serum lactate LDH >400 IU/l
     - serum AST >250 IU/l
     - hypoxaemia
     - low calcium (corrected for albumin).

Causes of acute pancreatitis

	Frequently encountered causes	**Less frequently encountered causes**
Cancer	Pancreatic cancer	Cancer of the ampulla of Vater
	Metastatic cancer to liver or porta hepatis	
Intercurrent illnesses	Gallstones	Post-ERCP
	Alcohol	Hypertriglyceridaemia
	Idiopathic	Medications (valproate, steroids, azathioprine, L-asparaginase)
		Infections (mumps, Coxsackie B, viral hepatitis)

History

- People present with a **sudden onset of pain**, which may be mild to very severe.
- The pain is localized to the **epigastrium** or may **radiate to the back** and lower abdomen.
- The pain is often relieved by sitting upright and bending forward.
- People may also experience **nausea and vomiting, anorexia, and fever**.
- There may be a change in bowel habits, progressing to a **paralytic ileus**.

Physical examination

- These individuals look unwell.
- Check **vital signs** and assess **hydration urgently**. They may be **febrile** and **shocked**.
- These people are often **agitated**.
- Abdominal examination may be unremarkable compared with the level of distress or may reveal a generally tender distended abdomen, with reduced or absent bowel sounds.
- Severe necrotizing pancreatitis can lead to tissue catabolism of haem giving **Cullen's sign** (peri-umbilical blue discoloration) and **Grey–Turner's sign** (flank discoloration).
- **Pleural effusions** may be present.

Investigations and management

Prognosis measured in hours to days prior to the onset of this problem (symptom control)

The **pain of pancreatitis may be very severe**. Although there have been concerns raised that morphine may exacerbate pain by causing spasm of the sphincter of Oddi, morphine is still the analgesia of choice. At this stage, this is best given via the subcutaneous route. The exception is if the person is shocked, when intravenous administration may be preferable.

People may have **nausea with vomiting**. This may be managed with metoclopramide (10 mg oral/SC/IV four times daily). The exception is in the presence of a paralytic ileus, in which case metoclopramide may be contraindicated. Alternative agents include haloperidol (0.5–3.0 mg oral/SC daily) and cyclizine (12.5–25 mg oral/SC three times daily).

Agitation secondary to pain, shock, hypoxaemia, infection, and possibly alcohol withdrawal may be seen. Although the prognosis is limited, it is imperative to consider a reversible cause of agitation (hypoxia, urinary retention, pain, fever) and gently reverse it. Simultaneously, agitation should be addressed with combinations of medications (haloperidol 0.5 mg hourly until settled and a benzodiazepine (diazepam 2.5–5.0 mg three times daily)).

Prognosis measured in weeks prior to the onset of this problem (in addition to symptom control)

- Although this is mostly a self-limiting disease, initially these people may be extremely unwell.
- **Fluid resuscitation, analgesia, antiemetics**, and treatment of **infection** are indicated.
- **If LFTs and ultrasound examination** confirm gallstone pancreatitis, urgent **ERCP** is indicated.
- If they have severe pancreatitis with no gallstones, transfer to a high dependency unit may not be appropriate.
- For prognostic purposes, a **biochemical assessment of severity** should be made by checking amylase, lipase, FBC, EUC, LFT, Ca, glucose, and LDH.

Prognosis measured in months to years prior to the onset of this problem (in addition to 'prognosis measured in weeks')

Investigations must include the following and should be initiated whilst obtaining a **high dependency opinion**:

- **serum amylase and lipase** are elevated (amylase >3–4 times the upper limit of normal)
- **renal function** (to help determine hydration status)
- liver function (looking for underlying pathology) with albumin
- **FBC** (anaemia, neutrophilia)
- **serum calcium** (corrected for albumin)
- **ABG**
- **LDH**
- a **plain abdominal and chest X-ray** are needed to exclude an acute abdomen secondary to perforation and to examine for an ileus
- an **abdominal ultrasound** will identify gallstones, any dilatation in the biliary tree, and any pseudocysts
- an **abdominal CT** will show loss of tissue planes around the pancreas in the presence of acute inflammation.
  The initial management includes:
- **urgent fluid resuscitation** (fluid sequestration) and careful monitoring; an indwelling urinary catheter should be inserted
- **opioid** analgesia is required
- **hourly monitoring** of vital signs and urine output
- **daily FBC, EUC, LFT, Ca, amylase, glucose, and ABG**.

The mortality of acute pancreatitis is estimated at 7–35 percent, with the majority of deaths occurring soon after diagnosis because of multi-organ failure. The remaining deaths are due to subsequent infection of the necrotic pancreas.

Further reading

Oxford Textbook of Medicine, Vol. 2, pp. 679–687.

:☹: Acute hepatocellular failure

- Acute liver failure is a syndrome of sudden hepatic dysfunction leading to encephalopathy, coagulopathy, circulatory collapse, renal failure, and infection.
- Acute hepatic failure is divided into hyperacute, acute, and subacute defined by the speed with which encephalopathy develops after the onset of jaundice.
- Mortality with fulminant hepatic failure is very high. The prognosis of acute liver failure is poor. In the presence of an infiltrating metastatic malignancy, mortality is 100 per cent. Other poor prognostic factors include rapidly developing jaundice, raised intracranial pressure, hypotension, sepsis, being HIV positive, or being elderly.

Causes of acute hepatic failure		
	Frequently encountered causes	**Less frequently encountered causes**
Cancer	Lymphoma	Malignant infiltration
Intercurrent illnesses	Acute viral hepatitis Autoimmune hepatitis	Other viruses (cytomegalovirus, Epstein–Barr virus)
		Budd–Chiari syndrome (hepatic vein thrombosis)
		Veno-occlusive disease of the liver
		Haemochromatosis
		Wilson's disease
Drugs	Paracetamol overdose	Halothane
		Isoniazid
		Antiretrovirals

History

People present with a **non-specific illness** of fatigue, nausea and vomiting, anorexia, and jaundice. The time course for these symptoms is usually very short. A thorough history of risk factors is necessary.

Physical examination

Physical examination may only disclose **new jaundice**. An estimate of **fluid status** is indicated, as these people may be severely dehydrated.

Neurological examination must be undertaken to exclude encephalopathy. Specifically test for asterixis, constructional apraxia, and a full Mini-Mental Status Examination (see Appendix 4).

These people are at risk of **cerebral oedema**, and should be observed for changes of hypertension, bradycardia, papillary changes, seizures, and decerebrate posturing.

The physical examination will allow the person to be graded as follows:
- grade 1: altered mood or behaviour
- grade 2: increasing drowsiness, confusion, slurred speech
- grade 3: stupor, incoherence, restlessness.

Investigations and management

Prognosis measured in hours to days prior to the onset of this problem (symptom control)

- These people will **deteriorate very rapidly**.
- **Nausea and vomiting** will require parenteral medications. Metoclopramide may be used.
- In an agitated person, haloperidol may be preferred.
- Consider cyclizine (12.5–25 mg SC four times daily) in a person with pruritus and jaundice.
- **Seizures** need to be addressed even in the terminal phases of care. Load with phenytoin (10–15 mg/kg by slow IV infusion, then continue 100 mg IV three times daily) and ensure a rescue dose of benzodiazepine (valium 5 mg IV or midazolam 5 mg SC) is available if seizures occur.
- If seizure activity persists despite these interventions, consider phenobarbital (100 mg SC loading dose, then 30 mg three times daily). Phenobarbital is useful in this situation as it causes cerebral vasoconstriction, is sedative, and is an antiepileptic.
- **Pain** due to inflammation of the hepatic capsule will require opioid analgesia.
- Even in the terminal stages, **dehydration** can cause significant symptoms, and gentle parenteral hydration will be of benefit.
- People who are **bleeding** should have vitamin K 10 mg IV daily. If there is any evidence of bleeding, these people must have crisis medications (p.52) available.
- The **jaundice may lead to itch**. In this group, it is reasonable to consider parenteral 5-HT$_3$ antagonists (ondansetron 4 mg SL/IV twice daily).

Prognosis measured in weeks prior to the onset of this problem (in addition to symptom control)

- The prognosis for fulminant hepatic failure in people with advanced life-limiting illness is extremely poor. **Poor prognostic factors include**:
  - grade III or IV encephalopathy
  - age >40 years
  - albumin <30 g/l
  - metastatic and drug-induced liver failure.
- Check **FBC, EUC, LFT, and albumin**.
- If **paracetamol overdose** is suspected, serum levels should be checked and treated with acetylcysteine.
- **Gentle hydration** with glucose-containing fluids should be continued.
- Do not allow the person to become constipated.

Prognosis measured in months to years prior to the onset of this problem (in addition to 'prognosis measured in weeks')
Few people with an established life-limiting illness will recover from fulminant hepatic failure. An urgent hepatology consultation must be sought to organize transfer to a high dependency unit. Transfer to a hepatobiliary unit provides the best chance of survival.

Investigations and management include the following:
- **LFTs** (elevated bilirubin, AST, ALT).
- **FBC** (infection, GI bleed).
- **Coagulation studies** (PT/INR).
- **Renal function** and **electrolytes**, BSL.
- **LDH.**
- **Viral serology.**
- **Serum paracetamol levels.**
- **Hepatic ultrasound**, looking specifically for Doppler flow in the hepatic and portal vasculature.
- High-resolution **spiral CT scan** may demonstrate miliary spread of malignancy to the liver.
- All **potentially hepatotoxic medications should be ceased**. Immediate treatment of reversible toxicity (paracetamol overdose) should be initiated.
- People who are developing an **encephalopathy** should be nursed in a quiet room, with the head of the bed elevated to 30°.
- Initiate oral or rectal **lactulose** to empty bowel and minimize encephalopathy.
- People who are **bleeding** should have vitamin K (10 mg IV daily for 3 days), platelets, and FFP
- **PPIs** should be commenced for all people.
- Carefully monitored **fluid resuscitation** is indicated as there is a 40–80 per cent incidence of associated renal failure (pre-renal, acute tubular necrosis, hepatorenal failure)
- There is **high risk of infection** (impaired complement synthesis), with incidence rates of 50 per cent for pneumonia and 30 per cent for urinary tract infections. Actively treat sepsis (initial antibiotic ceftriaxone 1 g IV/IM daily).
- **Hypoglycaemia** should be treated with 50 per cent glucose (glucagon alone will not be effective).

Further reading
Oxford Textbook of Medicine, Vol. 2, pp. 714–723.
Oxford Textbook of Palliative Medicine, pp. 507, 515–516.

⚙ Fistula formation

- A fistula is an abnormal opening connecting two hollow organs or a hollow organ and the skin.
- The most common acquired fistulae originate in the GI tract.
- Fistulae are associated with significant morbidity and mortality.

Causes of fistula formula*

	Frequently encountered causes	**Less frequently encountered causes**
Cancer	Any intra-abdominal malignancy	Previous radiotherapy
Intercurrent illnesses	Diverticulitis Inflammatory bowel disease Previous stenting	Pancreatitis Cholecystitis Appendicitis Trauma Previous abdominal surgery Ischaemic bowel Crohn's disease

*See also tracheo-oesophageal fistula (p.274)

History

The history depends on the site of the fistula.

- A fistula between the gut and the biliary system is often subclinical except when **gallstone ileus develops**. These people present with a history of nausea and vomiting consistent with small bowel obstruction.
- **Enterocutaneous fistulae** are typically preceded by an erythematous swelling. Once the fistula has developed, the diagnosis is very clear.
- Internal gut fistulae may be accompanied by a change in bowel habits, often with diarrhoea and pain.
- A **fistula between the pelvic organs and the gut** is accompanied by the passage of faecal matter or flatus when voiding or faecal matter through the vagina. This is often associated with incontinence (urinary and faecal), cystitis, and urinary tract infections.
- Rarely, **fistulae may develop between the upper gut and the vascular system**. This is rapidly fatal.

Physical examination

- The physical examination may be unremarkable.
- An already formed enterocutaneous fistula is obvious, with discharge of intestinal contents through the skin, often with surrounding cellulitis and excoriation.
- If the small bowel is involved, there is a significant risk that there will be dehydration.
- Examine the abdomen for any other localized tenderness or palpable mass as the pathology may be multifocal.

- For vaginal fistulae, inspect the perineal region for localized excoriation.
- Check temperature, pulse, and blood pressure (standing and sitting) for fluid status.

Investigations and management

Prognosis measured in hours to days prior to the onset of this problem (symptom control)

The **immediate priority** is to **control pain, infections, and dehydration**. Other interventions at this stage of life are to control the output from a fistula. This may be achieved by decreasing parenteral fluid intake and the use of octreotide (start with 100 µg SC three times daily).

People with enterocutaneous fistulae require review by a **specialist stoma therapy/wound care nurse** for the best application of drainage bags and to minimize skin problems, including autodigestion, and secondary bacterial and fungal infections.

There is a risk of **torrential bleeding** from fistulae, and crisis medications (p.52) must be readily available.

Prognosis measured in weeks prior to the onset of this problem (in addition to 'symptom control')

Investigations are dictated according to the presumed site of the fistula and the condition of the person.

For enterocutaneous fistulae, check **FBC, electrolytes** (there can be significant loss of K^+ and Na^+ in small bowel enterocutaneous fistulae), and renal function, and **assess the output** from the fistula.

For internal fistulae, **FBC (Hb, WCC), coagulation studies** (bleeding risk), **electrolytes, renal function, liver function, albumin, blood cultures**, and **urine cultures** (if febrile) are indicated.

Diagnosis of bowel-to-bowel fistulae can be difficult. Plain abdominal X-rays may be of no help, and contrast studies are sometimes difficult to interpret. A **gastrograffin study** should be done if a bowel-to-bowel fistula is suspected. An **abdominal CT** scan will give the most information about the location and cause of the fistula.

Endoscopy may be useful to assess whether or not stenting is possible especially for rectal lesions.

Surgical closure depends upon the location and the likelihood of cure. Malignant fistulae or fistulae at the site of previous radiotherapy are unlikely to gain good functional outcomes from surgical intervention.

Fistulae may be amenable to **palliative stenting** if the oesophagus, gastric outlet, duodenum, and rectum are involved.

Enterocutanous fistulae are usually accompanied by malnutrition, and there needs to be early consideration of parenteral feeding on a case-by-case basis.

Vitamin deficiencies need correction, especially if the distal small bowel is involved.

Octreotide may reduce outputs from enteric fistulae and assist with spontaneous closure.

*Prognosis measured in months to years prior to the onset of this
problem (in addition to 'prognosis measured in weeks')*
Mortality remains high as fistula formation is often evidence of progressive disease. Late diagnosis of internal fistulae significantly worsens outcomes.

Further reading

Oxford Textbook of Medicine, Vol. 2, pp. 501, 625–628.
Oxford Textbook of Palliative Medicine, pp. 258, 263, 638.
Oxford Handbook of Palliative Care, pp. 91–92.

☼ Sudden onset of jaundice

- Three main reasons for hyperbilirubinaemia are liver disease, obstruction of bile ducts, or isolated disorders of bilirubin metabolism.
- Jaundice is classified according to the type of circulating bilirubin (conjugated or unconjugated) or the site of the problem (pre-, intra- or post-hepatic).

Causes of a sudden onset of jaundice

	Frequently encountered causes	**Less frequently encountered causes**
Cancer	Nodes at the porta hepatis	Pancreatic carcinoma
	Hepatic metastases	Cholangiocarcinoma
Intercurrent illnesses	Gallstones	Sarcoidosis
	Gilbert's syndrome	Sickle cell crisis
	Shock	Haemolysis
	Septicaemia	Resorption of a haematoma
	Alcohol	
Drugs	Phenothiazines	Haloperidol
	Tricyclic antidepressants	Cyproheptadine
	Sulphonylureas	NSAIDs
	Penicillins	Phenytoin
		Carbamazepine
		Phenobarbital
		Thiazides
		Allopurinol
Spurious	Carrotonaemia (excessive carrot juice with sparing of the sclera)	

History
History must include recent infections, blood transfusions, medications (the list of medications causing cholestatsis, or cholestatic hepatitis is almost endless), and any previous episodes of jaundice.

A recent onset of fever associated with right upper quadrant pain (choledocolithiasis), and of fatigue, myalgia, and malaise (viral illness) must be sought.

Physical examination
- Check **temperature**, **blood pressure**, and **pulse rate** to estimate fluid status and infection.
- **Altered skin colour and scleral icterus** suggest serum bilirubin >35 mmol/l.
- **Scratch marks** reflect severe pruritus.

- Examine for tattoos and needle tracks, and peripheral stigmata of alcohol use (parotid enlargement, Dupytren's contracture, gynaecomastia).
- **Abdominal examination** includes trying to elicit Murphy's sign (p.148), liver size and contour, ascites, and bruising.
- Exclude splenomegaly and other evidence of **portal hypertension**.
- Auscultate over the liver for a **venous hum** (alcoholic hepatitis, hepatocellular cancer).
- Examine for **encephalopathy** (p.154).

Investigations and management
Prognosis measured in hours to days prior to the onset of this problem (symptom control)
People with **jaundice** have nausea (p.40) and pruritus. **Pruritus** in incomplete biliary obstruction may respond to cholestyramine. In complete obstruction use 5-HT$_3$ antagonists (ondansetron 4 mg SL or IV/SC twice daily) or paroxetine (20 mg daily). NB. Antihistamines are only useful in pruititis caused by urticaria and allergy.

Although these people are at the very end-of-life, dehydration should be treated to reduce itch.

Stop hepatoxic medications if possible.

Prognosis measured in weeks prior to the onset of this problem (in addition to 'symptom control')
Investigations include the following:
- **LFTs** (cholestatic, isolated elevated bilirubin, or globally impaired).
- **FBC** (anaemia, platelet count, reticulocyte count).
- **Blood film** (to suggest haemolysis).
- **Coagulation studies.**
- **Electrolytes and renal function.**
- Liver ultrasound looking for obstruction of the biliary free.
- Febrile people should have immediate blood cultures and it may be appropriate to commence intravenous hydration and antibiotics while awaiting the result (p.48).
- Any hepatoxic medications should be stopped.
- Treat hepatic encephalopathy if it is present (p.154).
- Cholestasis secondary to gallstones or malignant obstruction may be improved with an ERCP or percutaneous drainage of the biliary tree and, for malignant obstruction, stenting.

Prognosis measured in months to years prior to the onset of this problem (in addition to 'Prognosis measured in weeks')
Investigations are indicated to define the cause of the problem.
- Failure to reach a diagnosis based on preliminary screen indicates further investigations including **conjugated and unconjugated bilirubin estimation**.
- Cholestasis secondary to gallstones requires **endoscopic or surgical intervention**.

- Jaundice secondary to biliary duct compression (cancer, lymphoma) may be suitable for inserton of a **biliary stent**, with subsequent radiotherapy or chemotherapy in responsive cancers.
- **Hypoperfusion** and toxic liver damage require **supportive management** while avoiding further episodes of insult.
- Viral and autoimmune hepatic disease requires **specialist consultations**.

Further reading

Oxford Textbook of Medicine, Vol. 2, pp. 708–713.
Oxford Textbook of Palliative Medicine, pp. 507–512.
Oxford Handbook of Palliative Care, p. 92.

Haematological disorders

☠️ Neutropaenic sepsis

- Severe neutropenia is an absolute neutrophil count of $<0.5\times10^6/\mu l$. The risk of infection increases as the neutrophil count falls below $1.0\times10^6/\mu l$.
- Acute neutropenia is more often associated with bacterial infections while chronic neutropenia is associated with fungal infections.

Causes of neutropenia

Impaired production of neutrophils

- Drugs (cytotoxic chemotherapy, immunosuppressive therapy, sulfonamides, anti-thyroid medications, anticonvulsants)
- Post-infection
- Primary marrow failure especially with malignant infiltration
- Congenital (cyclic, congenital)

Nutritional deficiencies

Increased destruction of neutrophils

- Infection
- Immune-mediated destruction (SLE, rheumatoid arthritis with Felty's syndrome)
- Increased sequestration
- Splenomegaly

History

- A person with **acute neutropaenic** sepsis may fail to develop localizing signs except for fever or general influenza-like symptoms.
- A history of **recent cytotoxic chemotherapy** and **other drug history** must be sought.
- Check for **localizing symptoms of sepsis**. Chronic neutropenia is more likely to lead to chronic sinusitis or mouth ulcers.

Physical examination

People with neutropaenic sepsis may be febrile. Check for shock and hypo-thermia. Examine the mouth and ears, check for signs of meningism (photo-phobia, neck stiffness, and pain on straight leg raising (Kernig's sign)), examine chest and abdomen, palpate lymph nodes, palpate over the facial sinuses, and examine skin (including the perineum and injection sites (SC or IV)).

Investigations and management

Prognosis measured in hours to days prior to the onset of this problem (symptom control)

It is not appropriate to initiate further investigations in this group.

Treat fever and rigors:

- tepid sponges and control the ambient temperature
- regular paracetamol (1 g orally or 500 mg rectally four times daily) or NSAIDs (indomethacin 25 mg PO three times daily or 100 mg rectally twice daily or ketorolac 10 mg SC four times daily)
- consider a single dose of gentamicin 160 mg and ceftriaxone 1 g IV (or IM) as this may help settle fever.
- Ensure adequate hydration.

Prognosis measured in weeks to months (in addition to symptom control)
- Collect **FBC (with differential WCC)**, **blood cultures** (bacterial and fungal), and urine cultures.
- Review CXR to exclude pneumonia.
- If diarrhoea is present, ensure stool cultures are collected, microscopy requested, and stools are tested for *Clostridium difficile* toxin.
- Swab any wounds.
- Inspect intravenous catheter sites and take cultures through any central venous catheters.
- The three most important steps are:
  - suspension of myelosuppressive medications
  - prompt initiation of antibiotics
  - adequate fluid resuscitation.

The choice of antibiotic is dictated by local pathogens informing local practice. **Prolonged neutropenia** or **prior use of antibiotics** will increase the likelihood of fungal infections. A person **without a spleen** (either surgically or functionally) must be covered for capsulated organisms (*Streptococcus pneumoniae*, *Haemophilus influenzae*, *Neisseria meningitis*). Infectious disease review should be sought in people with fever failing to resolve in 72 hs. A person who is haemodynamically stable, who can swallow, and who is expected to have normal absorption may be managed with oral antibiotics. Otherwise, use parenteral therapy.

Growth factors (G-CSF, GM-CSF) are used in cytotoxic-induced neutropaenia and in some people with chronic neutropaenia (congenital, cyclic autoimmune, or HIV/AIDS). These agents reduce the period of neutropenia, but do not reduce mortality.

Autoimmune neutropaenia may require regular corticosteroids and intermittent growth factor injections.

Prognosis measured in months to years prior to the onset of this problem (in addition to above)
Further investigations will be necessary if the source of sepsis is not identified. These include a **CT of the facial sinuses, high-resolution CT of the chest** looking for fungal infections, **echocardiogram**, and **bone marrow examination**.

The risk of mortality for people with acute neutropenia is about 7 per cent. Factors predicting poorer outcomes include continuing haemodynamic instability, organ failure, fever lasting more than 6 days, and gut or intravenous line infections.

Further reading
Oxford Textbook of Medicine, Vol. 3, pp. 586–588.
Oxford Textbook of Palliative Medicine, p. 867.
Oxford Handbook of Palliative Care, pp. 291–292, 763–764.

:☠: Disseminated intravascular coagulation

- DIC is a syndrome characterized by the loss of control of intravascular coagulation resulting in thrombosis and bleeding.
- DIC doubles the mortality of the underlying condition.

Causes of DIC

	Frequently encountered causes	**Less frequently encountered causes**
Cancer	Haematological malignancy	Carcinoid
	Adenocarcinomas	Sarcoma
Intercurrent illnesses	Pancreatitis	Fat embolism (bone fracture, crush injury)
	Sepsis	Aortic aneurysms
End-stage organ failure	Hepatic failure	
	Graft versus host disease	

History

People are often already **seriously unwell** from the medical condition that underlies the DIC. They will develop **bleeding** from any site and **extensive bruising**. At any point **thrombosis** may cause organ failure or gangrene.

Physical examination

People may have widespread **bruising and bleeding** from mucous membranes, intravenous catheter sites, wounds, and indwelling catheters.
They may have impaired blood supply to the digits, nose, and ear lobes because of fibrin deposition, resulting in ischaemic skin ulcers.

Investigations and management

Prognosis measured in hours to days prior to the onset of this problem (symptom control)

- **The symptoms and signs of DIC demand good palliation.**
- The most severe implication of DIC is the occurrence of **organ failure secondary to microthrombi.**
- Symptoms must be considered and managed as necessary. It is likely that people will require:
  - **analgesia** (digital and visceral infarcts, internal bleeding, PE)
  - management of **delirium** (organ failure, CNS microthrombi)
  - management of other symptoms which may include increasing **shortness of breath** (PE, anaemia), anxiety, and **nausea and vomiting** (organ failure, internal bleeding, gut ischaemia).
- Although the risk of catastrophic bleeding is low, it is necessary to ensure that **crisis medications** (p.52) are available.

- Platelet half-life in DIC is short, and platelet transfusion is unlikely to be of prolonged benefit.
- Mouth care with tranexamic acid solution as a mouthwash (1 g orally four times daily) may reduce oozing from oral mucosa.

Prognosis measured in weeks prior to the onset of this problem (in addition to symptom control)

Treatment of the underlying cause is the only definitive treatment of DIC. Consideration must be given to the cause of the DIC and whether or not this is likely to be reversible in this group of people.

Investigations include:
- **FBC** (low Hb, low platelets).
- **blood film** (fragmented red cells).
- **coagulation studies** (prolonged PT, APPT, decreased fibrinogen).
- markedly increased **D-dimer** (product of fibrin degeneration).

Supportive measures to address DIC include the following:
- Administration of **vitamin K** 10 mg orally or IV.
- Cryoprecipitate should be given only if fibrinogen is low.
- FFP should be given to correct coagulation but it also replaces antithrombin III, protein C and protein S.
- **Platelets** may occasionally be given for clinically serious bleeding as short-term salvage, but are otherwise contraindicated.
- Although the net benefit of heparin in DIC has yet to be proven in clinical trials, it may be used in clinically significant thrombus. This should be discussed with a haematologist.

Prognosis measured in months to years prior to the onset of this problem (in addition to the above)

Some people, especially with malignancy, may have low-grade DIC with which they coexist over long periods of time.

Further reading

Oxford Textbook of Medicine, Vol. 3, pp. 753–754, 70.
Oxford Handbook of Palliative Care, pp. 400–403.

☼ Thrombocytopaenia

- Thrombocytopaenia is a reduction in platelets to less than 150×10^9/l.
- Spontaneous bleeding generally does not occur until the platelet count is 10×10^9/L or less, or function is affected.
- Bleeding with trauma may occur with counts less than 40×10^9/l.

Causes of low platelet counts

	Frequently encountered causes	Less frequently encountered causes
Decreased production	Bone marrow metastases	Myelodysplasia
	Haematological malignancies	Toxic (alcohol)
		Folate/B$_{12}$ deficiency
		Paroxysmal nocturnal haemoglobinuria
Increased destruction	ITP	Drug-induced
	Lymphoproliferative disorders	Evans' syndrome
	HIV	DIC
	SLE	TTP
	Antiphospholipid antibodies	HUS
	Sepsis	Malignant hypertension
	Hypersplenism	
Increased sequestration	Splenomegaly	Hypothermia
	Cardiopulmonary bypass	
	Haemodilution	

Causes of impaired platelet function

Frequently encountered causes	Less frequently encountered causes
NSAIDs including aspirin, clopidogrel, ticlopidine	Marrow failure
	Myelodysplasia
	Renal failure

History

A **drug history** includes recent use of heparin, antibiotics (rifampicin, trimethoprim, sulphur-containing medications), cardiac medications (quinine, procainamide, thiazide diuretics), and RA-modifying agents.

Check for recent blood transfusions or surgery, fever, arthralgia, a diagnosis of HIV (or risk factors), and heavy alcohol use.

☼ Anaemia

- Adults are anaemic when the haemoglobin concentration is <13.0 g/dl in men and <11.5 g/dl in women.
- Acute anaemia is caused by blood loss or rapid haemolysis.

Causes of anaemia	
Blood loss	Erosion of a major blood vessel
	Failure of normal haemostasis
	Surgery
	Trauma
	GIT blood loss
Haemolysis	Inherited disorders
	Hereditary spherocytosis or elliptocytosis
	Red cell enzyme defects
	Acquired disorders
	Hypersplenism
	Warm antibody
	idiopathic, lymphoma, drugs,
	collagen vascular disorders
	Cold antibody
	infection, idiopathic, lymphoma,
	paroxysmal cold haemoglobinuria
Ineffective haemopoesis	Reduced red cell production due to bone marrow infiltration
	multiple myeloma, prostate cancer, breast cancer, leukaemia
	Chemotherapy-induced marrow suppression
	Nutritional (either inadequate intake or malabsorption of vitamin B_{12}, folate, iron)
	Reduced erythropoietin
	chronic renal failure
Other	Anaemia of chronic disease

History

- Anaemia causes **fatigue, increasing shortness of breath on exertion, angina, palpitations, headache, impaired concentration, anorexia,** and **weakness.**
- People may describe **symptoms of heart failure** (orthopnoea, PND, and increasing ankle oedema).
- Check for a **history of bleeding** (rectal, vaginal, haematuria).
- Check the **drug history** (NSAIDs, aspirin, heparin, warfarin).

Physical examination

- Check for **pallor of the palmar creases** and **pale conjunctiva**. There may be a tachycardia.
- If the cause of the anaemia is blood loss, the **pulse may be thready** and the person may be **hypotensive**. Alternatively, there may be a **hyperdynamic state** with cardiac enlargement (in chronic anaemia) and flow murmurs leading to cardiac failure.
- Examine for **signs of bleeding**, including a rectal examination.

Investigations and management

Prognosis measured in days to hours prior to the onset of this problem (symptom control)

This is a clinical diagnosis based on history and appearance. Medications that may contribute to blood loss should be discontinued if possible.

Active bleeding should be addressed by local measures (tranexamic acid mouthwashes, local pressure, and epinephrine-soaked sponges). Consider an infusion of packed cells if dyspnoea or clouded cognition is causing distress and a primary site of bleeding can be identified and controlled. If the person is at risk of, or clinically in heart failure, the transfusion should proceed slowly with furosemide 20–40 mg IV/SC cover. The dose will depend upon previous use of this medication and any past history of renal dysfunction. Ensure that crisis medications (p.52) are available.

Prognosis measured in weeks prior to the onset of this problem (in addition to symptom control)

The initial investigations include a full blood count and **examination of the blood film**. This allows the anaemia to be classified into:
- microcytic (MCV <80 fl)
- normocytic (MCV 80–100 fl)
- macrocytic (MCV >100 fl).

A **microcytic anaemia** is most likely to be due to:
- iron deficiency, increased RDW, anisocytosis, poikilocytosis, thrombocytosis
- anaemia of chronic disease
- thalassaemia (polychromasia, target cells).

The **ferritin level** will be low in iron deficiency and normal to high in chronic disease or with any inflammatory process. Transfuse packed cells if the person is symptomatic. If tolerated, oral iron may be commenced.

A **normocytic anaemia** may occur in people who have:
- active bleeding
- anaemia associated with chronic disease including renal failure
- haemolysis (spherocytes, schistocytes, bite cells)
- marrow failure (abnormal differential count, blast cells, dimorphic blood cells, Pelger–Huet cells, rouleaux).

People **actively bleeding** require stabilization (local control, fluid re-suscitation). Check **coagulation studies** and administer packed cells and, if necessary, FFP and platelets. If bleeding is not controlled, **consider surgical or radiological review** to provide haemostasis. A person with anaemia from chronic disease is best managed supportively.

A haemolytic screen includes LDH (raised), **haptoglobins** (raised), **indirect bilirubin** (very high), and **reticulocyte count** (low).

Haemolysis may occur secondary to genetic disorders including:
• red cell membrane disorders (e.g. hereditary spherocytosis)
• haemoglobin disorders (e.g. sickle cell anaemia, thalassaemia)
• enzyme defects (e.g. glucose-6-phosphate dehydrogenase deficiency).

Causes of acquired haemolysis include the following
• Immune:
  • isoimmune (blood transfusion reaction)
  • autoimmune (warm or cold autoantibodies)
  • drug reaction (penicillin, a-methyldopa, mefenamic acid, or l -dopa)
• Non-immune:
  • trauma (prosthetic heart valve, microangiopathic secondary to HUS)
  • septicaemia
  • membrane disorders (paroxysmal nocturnal haemoglobinuria, liver disease).
  • previous episodes or a family history of haemolysis should identify familial causes.

Known precipitants to genetic haemolysis include medications (ciprofloxacin, sulphonamides, primaquine), infections, and dehydration. Management is supportive. Discontinue new medications, maintain hydration, and provide analgesia.

In people with warm autoimmune haemolytic anaemia, a trial of steroids is indicated. Cold autoimmune haemolytic anaemia typically presents with a symptomatic anaemia and Raynaud's syndrome in cold weather, and is best managed by ensuring that the person is nursed in a warm ambient temperature.

A **macrocytic anaemia** with increased RDW may be due to the following:
• Medications (oval macrocytes: zidovudine, hydroxyurea).
• Nutritional (increased RDW, oval macrocytes):
  • thiamine deficiency
  • folate deficiency
  • vitamin B_{12} deficiency.
• Myelodysplasia or marrow infiltration (dimorphic blood cells).
• Liver disease (normal RDW, round macrocytes).
• Hypothyroidism (normal RDW, round macrocytes).
• Bone marrow failure (abnormal differential count, blast cells, dimorphic blood cells, Pelger–Huet cells, rouleaux).

Thiamine deficiency may present with neurological abnormalities (confusion, ataxia, ophthalmoplegia, nystagmus) and cardiac dysfunction (general oedema, biventricular failure). Commence thiamine replacement with 100 mg orally or IV daily.

Vitamin B_{12} deficiency may present with subacute combined degeneration of the spinal cord. This affects the posterior and/or lateral columns. Onset is slow. A peripheral neuropathy occurs, with joint position and vibration sense the first to be affected. Later, sensory changes with increasing weakness and stiffness occur. It is reasonable to replace B_{12}

with cyanocobalamin 1000 µg/ml IM daily for 3 days and then reduce to once a month.

Bone marrow failure may be due to stem cell failure (aplastic anaemia occurring secondary to drugs, viral hepatitis, autoimmune causes, inherited causes, and cytotoxic therapy), malignant infiltration, or myelodysplasia. These people require transfusion support and treatment of infections. Discontinue medications that may have precipitated this problem (chemotherapy agents, gold).

Further reading

Oxford Textbook of Medicine, Vol. 3, p. 501.
Oxford Textbook of Palliative Medicine, pp. 568, 603.
Oxford Handbook of Palliative Care, pp. 391–398.

Hyperviscosity

- Blood viscosity is a function of the concentration of the plasma and the make-up of blood components.
- Its clinical manifestation is due to impaired microcirculation.

Causes of hyperviscosity

	Frequently encountered causes	**Less frequently encountered causes**
Cancer	Myeloma	CML, CLL, AML
Intercurrent illnesses	Polycythaemia secondary to COPD	Primary polycythaemia Waldenstrom's macroglobulinaemia

History

A history of **headaches, blurred vision**, and **increasing confusion** may be present. In severe cases, **cerebral ischaemia** presents with vertigo, ataxia, and diplopia. People may describe **increasing shortness of breath** and **chest pain**. Additionally, a person may describe haematuria, rectal bleeding, or melaena.

Physical examination

- There may be **digital infarcts**.
- Examine for **nystagmus, gait disorder**, and **impaired Mini Mental Status Examination** (see Appendix 4). Examination should also include **funduscopy** for retinal vein engorgement or flame-shaped haemorrhages.
- Check for signs of **left ventricular failure** and **tender hepatosplenomegaly**.

Investigations and management

Prognosis measured in hours to days prior to the onset of this problem (symptom control)

Although the prognosis is short, ensuring **adequate hydration** may improve comfort.

Prognosis measured in weeks to months prior to the onset of this problem (in addition to symptom control)

- **FBC with a blood film** will identify polycythaemia or leukocytosis. Bone marrow examination is not indicated. Check **renal function and coagulation factors**.
- Ensure adequate hydration.
- **Plasmapheresis** may be necessary to keep the symptoms of hyperviscosity under control in people who are too unwell for definitive treatment.

Prognosis measured in months to years prior to the onset of this problem (in addition to the above)

Seek definitive treatment of the cause. If active disease-modifying measures have been exhausted, symptomatic support is based on optimizing renal function and hydration in myeloma, and in reducing viscosity with plasmapheresis in hyperleukocytosis.

Further reading

Oxford Textbook of Medicine, Vol. 2, p. 1081; Vol. 3, p. 621.

☼ Sickle cell crisis

- The inherited haemoglobin variants responsible for sickling crises are HbSS, HbSC, HbS/beta thalassaemia, and HbSD.
- Haemoglobin S forms polymers when deoxygenated, which causes the normally pliable red blood cells to become stiff and crescent shaped, clogging capillaries and leading to veno-occlusion and tissue hypoxia necrosis.

Precipitants of sickle cell crisis
Hypoxaemia
Infection
Dehydration
Temperature extremes
Physical stress
Psychological stress

History

The major symptom is **pain**, which may be localized or diffuse. The pain is generally associated with **fever, and nausea and vomiting**. There may be **increased shortness of breath, pleuritic chest pain, joint swelling**, and the development of **leg ulcers**.

Physical examination

- Check **temperature** and **other vital signs**.
- Perform a peripheral examination for stigmata of **anaemia, digital infarcts**, or **leg ulcers**.
- Perform a **neurological examination** to seek evidence of cerebral ischaemia.
- Check for **hepatosplenomegaly** and ensure that **priapism** is not present.

Investigations and management

Prognosis measured in hours to days prior to the onset of this problem (symptom control)

Even in this group, management includes **adequate hydration and analgesia**. This should be opioids (either continuous by PCA or IV). Sickle cell crisis may require significant doses of opioid even in the opioid-naive person. Consider addition of NSAIDs (ketorolac 10 mg SC four times daily) and paracetamol. **Oxygen** is only indicated with hypoxaemia.

Maintain an **even temperature** and do not allow the person to become cold.

Prognosis measured in weeks prior to the onset of this problem (in addition to symptom control)

Check FBC (anaemia, increased WCC, platelet count may be either increased or decreased, increased reticulocyte count). Check **renal and liver function**, especially for bilirubin levels. Check **pulse oximetry** and **arterial blood gases** looking for hypoxaemia. Regardless of whether or not the person is febrile, a **septic screen** is indicated, including a **CXR** and **blood cultures**. An **ECG** is indicated if there is chest pain.

A broad-spectrum antibiotic should be added, even without the results of a septic screen (functional hyposplenism). Maintain an even temperature and do not allow the person to become cold. Exchange transfusion may be necessary in the presence of priapism, cerebral ischaemia, or cardiac ischaemia.

Further reading

Oxford Textbook of Medicine, Vol. 3, pp. 690–691, 1484–1485.
Oxford Textbook of Palliative Medicine, p. 845.

Metabolic disorders

☼ Acute renal failure

- Acute renal failure refers to an acute (hours to days) deterioration in the glomerular filtration rate leading to an accumulation of nitrogenous waste products (creatinine and urea).
- This is commonly (although not universally) associated with decreasing urine output, sometimes leading to anuria.
- As a result, fluid balance, electrolyte balance, and acid–base balance are impaired.
- The causes of acute renal failure are grouped according to aetiology:
  - pre-renal failure (underperfused kidneys)
  - post-renal failure (compression of the collecting system)
  - intrinsic renal failure
  - decompensated (or acute-or-chronic) chronic renal failure.

Causes of acute renal failure

	Frequently encountered causes	**Less frequently encountered causes**
Pre-renal failure	Hypoperfusion (haemorrhage, volume depletion)	
	Inadequate effective vascular volumes (heart failure, hypoalbuminaemia, ascites)	
	Acute disruption to renal artery blood flow	
	Drugs that interfere with GFR and renal blood flow (ACE inhibitors, angiotensin II inhibitors, NSAIDs)	
Post-renal failure	Obstruction of the collecting system (bladder outlet obstruction, uretric obstruction)	
Intrinsic renal failure	Acute tubular necrosis (ischaemic, gentamicin, radio-contrast, cisplatin, uric acid, myoglobinuria, haemo-globinuria, HUS, TTP)	Vasculitis Acute interstitial nephritis Glomerular nephritis Malignant hypertension Hepatorenal syndrome
Decompensated chronic renal failure	Glomerular nephritis Pyelonephritis Interstitial nephritis Diabetic nephropathy Hypertensive nephropathy Polycystic kidney disease Analgesic nephropathy Renovascular disease Nephrolithiasis	Myeloma Amyloidosis SLE Scleroderma Gout Vasculitis Haemolytic uraemic syndrome Renal tumours

History

Pre-renal failure may present with symptoms associated with diminished fluid reserve. These people may have **thirst, symptoms of postural hypotension, dry mouth**, and **sensation of anxiousness and unease**, which is often associated with bleeding.

A recent **change in medications** (ACE inhibitors, angiotensin II inhibitors, NSAIDs), recent radiology studies, or recent chemotherapy should be sought.

A history of acute deterioration and rapid changes in blood pressure should be sought from staff who have previously been caring for this person (ischaemic acute tubular necrosis, pre-renal failure).

Difficulties passing urine, nocturia, haematuria, and **flank pain** radiating **to the groin suggest an obstructive cause.**

A past history of chronic renal failure and recent changes that may account for this acute deterioration should be sought. In this group, check for any recent changes to medications (NSAIDs, ACE inhibitors, angiotensin II inhibitors, diuretics, lithium, cyclosporin). Check also for symptoms to suggest obstruction (difficulty voiding, haematuria), infection (fever, sweats, dysuria), hypercalcaemia, and hyperglycaemia.

As people become more unwell with **uraemia**, they will become drowsy, nauseated and confused. Eventually, they may develop seizures.

Physical examination

- Check **pulse, blood pressure** (include postural blood pressure), **pulse oximetry**, and **temperature**. Check for visible signs of bleeding, bruising, and anaemia.
- Examine for a **flap**. Check the skin for **scratch marks** (uraemic itch) and palpable purpura of **vasculitis**.
- **Cardiovascular** and **respiratory examination** includes an assessment of fluid status (JVP tissue turgor, pulmonary oedema, peripheral and sacral oedema, pleural effusions). Auscultate the heart for a **pericardial rub**.
- Palpate the abdomen for **ascites**. Check for **ballotable renal masses** and percuss for a bladder.
- There may be **muscle weakness** or **muscle paralysis** in the presence of severe **hyperkalaemia**.
- Include a neurological **assessment of mental state**.

Investigations and management

Prognosis measured in hours to days prior to the onset of this problem (symptom control)

- Despite the poor prognosis of this group, an **assessment of their fluid status** should be made. **Nephrotoxic medications** should be stopped and the dosage of medications that are renally excreted should be modified.
- People who are **fluid overloaded** and in pulmonary oedema require oxygen, diuretics (furosemide 40–80 mg IV/SC) (if not anuric), and morphine (2.5–5.0 mg SC/IV in the opioid naive).
- In people who are **fluid depleted**, rehydration with either SC or IV fluids is indicated (0.9 per cent NaCl 1 in 8–10 hs). This must be reviewed frequently as eventually the ability to tolerate the fluid load may become impaired.
- Other problems of increasing uraemia at the end-of-life will need to be palliated.
  - **Nausea**: haloperidol 0.5–3.0 mg SC daily. Alternatives include cyclizine 12.5–25 mg SC twice to four times daily and ondansetron 4–8 mg SL once or twice daily.
  - **Itch**: ondansetron 4–8 mg SL twice daily. Ensure that the skin is not dry and use regular moisturizers (Sorbolene cream).
  - **Myoclonic jerks**: clonazepam 0.5 mg SC/SL twice daily.

- **Breathlessness**: morphine 2.5 mg SC. Initially administer every 6–8 hs and titrate to response).
- **Dry mouth** with halitosis from uraemic saliva: institute regular mouth care.

Prognosis measured in weeks prior to the onset of this problem (in addition to symptom control)

Check **FBC** and **coagulation studies** (including bleeding time), **EUC, LFT, albumin, BSL, and calcium**. The aim is both to assess the severity of renal impairment and to identify factors that can easily be reversed in this population. It is unlikely that this group would be considered for dialysis.

Immediate life-threatening problems that need to be considered and addressed include the following:

- **Pulmonary oedema**: management of this problem includes sitting the person upright. Administer oxygen, diuretics, and morphine, and apply a glyceryl trinitrate patch (25–50 mg depending on the blood pressure). People who are very frightened by this breathlessness may require an anxiolytic medication (lorazepam 0.5–1.0 mg SL).
- **Hyperkalaemia**: organize an ECG. Changes of hyperkalaemia include tenting of the T wave, reduced height of the P wave, widening of the QRS, and increased PR interval. If the potassium is elevated biochemically but the ECG is normal, the first step should be intravenous administration of 50 ml of 50% glucose and rapidly acting insulin (actrapid 10 U) over 10 min. This should be followed by either oral or rectal sodium or calcium polystyrene sulphonate (Resonium 15 mg orally or 15–30 mg rectally). If there are ECG changes, the initial step should be 10 ml of intravenous 10% calcium carbonate to stabilize the cardiac membranes.
- **Bleeding**: acute bleeding may be the precipitating problem that may be exacerbated by the uraemic state. These people require fluid resuscitation and administration of packed cells and platelets. Desmopressin 0.3 U/kg IV will help prolong bleeding time.

Once these acute issues have been addressed, attention will need to be paid to:

- maintenance of fluid balance
- avoidance of nephrotoxic medications
- dose modifications of renally excreted medications
- treatment of underlying problems such as hyperglycaemia and hypercalcaemia
- correcting or preventing urinary tract obstruction.

Prognosis measured in months to years prior to the onset of this problem (in addition to the above)

The investigations and management of these people is best approached in a stepwise fashion. First, complications should be treated.

- Treat hyperkalaemia.

- **Pulmonary oedema**: organize a CXR, EUC, FBC, and ECG. Treat with diuretics, morphine, and nitrates. Administer oxygen. Consult high dependency services for transfer to coronary care if not settling.
- **Bleeding**: check FBC, coagulation studies including bleeding time. Insert a large-bore cannula and commence fluid resuscitation. Administer packed cells, platelets, and desmopressin. Seek a surgical consultation.
- Once these acute problems have been stabilized, the precipitating factor should be sought and addressed if possible.
- **Hypovolaemia** (dehydration, overdiuresis, bleeding, ineffective systemic circulation)
  - sepsis
  - cardiac failure
  - urinary obstruction.

A renal consultation should be sought to ascertain whether or not dialysis is indicated in this person. Indications for dialysis include:
  - persistent hyperkalaemia or disordered acid–base balance
  - uraemic encephalopathy
  - pericarditis
  - refractory pulmonary oedema.

Oliguric renal failure carries a better prognosis than anuric renal failure.

Further reading

Oxford Textbook of Medicine, Vol. 3 pp. 248–262, 263–278.
Oxford Textbook of Palliative Medicine, p. 698–699.
Oxford Handbook of Palliative Care, pp. 218–221, 314.

☠ Hyperkalaemia

- A low-level increase in serum potassium will be asymptomatic.
- Higher levels are an emergency which can cause premature mortality.

Causes of hyperkalaemia

	Frequently encountered causes	**Less frequently encountered causes**
Cancer		Tumour lysis syndrome
Intercurrent illnesses	Renal failure, potassium-sparing diuretics (spironolactone, triamterene, amiloride), hypoaldosteronism (ACE inhibitors, angiotensin II receptor blockade ('…statins'), NSAIDs, tacrolimus, cyclosporin, Addison's disease)	Rhabdomyolysis, digoxin toxicity and beta-blockers (redistribute K^+ to the extracellular space), any cause of acidosis

History

For most people, hyperkalaemia is an **incidental finding** associated with mild uraemia. In anyone with hyperkalaemia, review the medication list and recent history of fluid intake. **Muscle weakness** presenting as fatigue should prompt review of serum potassium. The most serious complications is **cardiac arrhythmias.**

Physical examination

Physical examination will most often be normal. Check **hydration status** to exclude hypovolaemia as a pre-renal cause of kidney impairment. Exclude **muscle injury** due to prolonged immobility (the person not found for prolonged periods after a fractured neck of femur or after a cerebrovascular accident).

Investigations and management

Prognosis measured in hours to days prior to the onset of this problem (symptom control)
No change to comfort care should be initiated unless the person is symptomatically dehydrated (beyond just a dry mouth).

Prognosis measured in weeks prior to the onset of this problem (in addition to 'prognosis measured in hours')
Establish the underlying cause. Stop any medications that may be contributing to the problem. Hydrate in renal failure secondary to decreased oral intake. Consider use of cation exchange resins which can bring potassium down within 1–2 hs (oral or rectal Resonium 15–30 gm two or three times daily). Ensure a **baseline** ECG is done. 'Sine wave' ECG is a late manifestation hyperkalaemia and is immediately life threatening.

Prognosis measured in months to years prior to the onset of this problem (in addition to 'prognosis measured in weeks')

In this population, consider an insulin–glucose infusion (50 U of actrapid in 50 ml 50% dextrose run IV at 5 ml/h initially) which will start to lower potassium within 30 min. In critically high levels, consider immediate dialysis.

Further reading

Oxford Textbook of Medicine, Vol. 3, p. 220

① **Hypokalaemia**

Causes of hypokalaemia

	Frequently encountered causes	**Less frequently encountered causes**
Intercurrent illnesses	Vomiting, diarrhoea, diuretics (except those that cause K^+ retention), diabetic ketoacidosis	Renal tubular acidosis, causes of acute metabolic or respiratory alkalosis, primary hyperaldosteronism, fludrocortisone excess, β_2 adrenergic excess.

History

This is almost certainly an incidental laboratory finding. Take a thorough medication history.

Weakness and fatigue should raise the question of **hypokalaemia**. New-onset polyuria or polydipsia can be a symptom of renal tubular dysfunction. GIT symptoms can include the first presentation of an ileus, and hypokalaemia needs to be in the differential consideration of constipation. In severe hypokalaemia, rhabdomyolysis may occur.

Physical examination

Physical examination will most often be normal. Check **hydration status** if vomiting or diarrhoea are the likely cause of low potassium. Check cardiac function. Check for muscle tenderness.

Investigations and management

Prognosis measured in hours to days prior to the onset of this problem
Continue to focus on comfort measures. Hypokalaemia will be asymptomatic in this population.

Prognosis measured in weeks or more prior to the onset of this problem (in addition to 'prognosis measured in hours')
Establish the underlying cause. Obtain a baseline **ECG**. **Replace potassium orally** unless the person is unable to tolerate oral administration.

Further reading

Oxford Textbook of Medicine, Vol. 3, pp. 213–219.

☹ **Hyponatraemia**

- Symptomatic hyponatraemia can occur with serum sodium below 125 mmol/l.
- The speed of onset of the hyponatraemia will dictate the speed of the response. Acute drops need to be treated actively in appropriate people because ensuing acute cerebral oedema will be fatal.

Causes of hyponatraemia

	Frequently encountered causes	**Less frequently encountered causes**
Cancer		Ascites or pleural effusions*
Other life-limiting illnesses	End-stage cardiac failure[‡] Cirrhosis[‡] Renal failure[‡]	
Intercurrent illnesses	Diuretics* Vomiting or diarrhoea* Pancreatitis Peritonitis*	SIADH[†] Addison's disease[†] Hypothyroidism[†] Nephrotic syndrome[‡] Hyperglycaemia*

* Salt loss greater than water loss.
[†] Normal total body water content.
[‡] Water retention greater than salt retention.

History

Hyponatraemia needs to be considered in people with a change in level of consciousness or impaired mentation. Lethargy may be a prominent symptom for some people. It is a frequently encountered cause of an **acute confusional state** (p. 28). Check serum sodium in anyone presenting with seizure activity (for the first time or with **seizure activity** that has become unstable).

Physical examination

Careful assessment of **hydration** is the key to categorizing hyponatraemia. Assess for **oedema** (cardiac in origin or nephrotic syndrome), but also ensure that there is no dehydration from vomiting or diarrhoea. Establish cognition and record the baseline mental state with the Mini Mental Status Examination (Appendix 4) Examine for evidence of cardiac failure or third-space relocation (pleural effusions or ascites). Seek signs of hypothyroidism.

Investigations and management

Prognosis measured in hours to days prior to the onset of this problem (symptom control)

In the last few hours of life, **treat symptoms directly**. If fluid overloaded and symptomatic, consider a loop diuretic. If hyponatraemia is severe, consider clonazepam 0.5 g–1 mg daily as an antiepileptic.

Prognosis measured in weeks prior to the onset of this problem in addition to 'prognosis measured in hours'

Establish the likely causes of hyponatraemia. If fluid overloaded, establish a fluid restriction and consider a regular loop diuretic. Stop medications that can cause hyponatraemia. If this includes diuretics, ensure that this is done with care so as not to worsen cardiac failure. If there is no oedema, check thyroid function tests, and if there is hyperkalaemia consider an ACTH level which will be raised in Addison's disease so that glucocorticoid replacement can be considered.

Prognosis measured in months to years prior to the onset of this problem (in addition to 'prognosis measured in weeks')

Careful evaluation of the causes of underlying cardiac or renal failure need to be explored and treated.

Further reading

Oxford Textbook of Palliative Medicine, p. 693.
Oxford Handbook of Palliative Care, pp. 424–429.

Syndrome of inappropriate antidiuretic hormone secretion (SIADH)

- SIADH is a dilutional hyponatraemia as ADH (vasopressin) continues to be produced despite low serum osmolality (no response to the negative feedback loop to downregulate ADH secretion).
- SIADH is a diagnosis of exclusion.

Causes of SIADH

	Frequently encountered causes	Less frequently encountered causes
Cancer	Small cell lung carcinoma	Mesothelioma
	Pancreatic carcinomas	Cyclophosphamide
	Any CNS tumour	Vincristine
		Vinblastine
Intercurrent illnesses	Pneumonia (or any chest infection)	Meningitis
	Tricyclic antidepressants	Intracranial bleed
	Haloperidol	Hypothyroidism
	Thiazide diuretics	Chlorpropamide
		MAOIs

History

Most SIADH is related to cerebral or intrathoracic pathology. It is difficult to make the diagnosis of SIADH in the presence of widespread oedema or medications known to be a direct cause of salt depletion. Review all the medications that the person is receiving and check for non-prescribed medications. As a diagnosis of exclusion, a history of thyroid dysfunction and autoimmune problems that could be associated with Addison's disease need to be explored. Exclude meningitis.

Physical examination

Physical examination will often be normal with absence of oedema. Exclude hypotension. Exclude signs of pneumonia or meningitis. Carefully evaluate the person's mental state.

Investigations and management

Prognosis measured in hours to days prior to the onset of this problem (symptom control)
Hyponatraemia in this setting should not be acted on. Minimize the risk of fitting with severe hyponatraemia (p. 210).

Prognosis measured in weeks prior to the onset of this problem in addition to 'prognosis measured in hours'
Establish the diagnosis (low serum sodium, low serum osmolality, high urinary sodium (often >30 mmol/l), urinary osmolality >100 mosmol/kg (but urine not maximally dilute) and hypouricaemia) and the underlying

cause. Check renal and thyroid function before making the diagnosis. If there is hypokalaemia, check ACTH levels before making the diagnosis of SIADH.

Review the benefit of medications that may be causing SIADH and stop them if appropriate. If there is CNS sepsis, treat aggressively with appropriate antibiotics (p. 48). Restrict fluid to 1000 ml/day and watch sodium levels regularly.

Prognosis measured in months to years prior to the onset of this problem (in addition to 'prognosis measured in weeks')

In people not responding adequately to fluid restriction, it is reasonable to induce nephrogenic diabetes insipidus with oral demethylchlortetracycline (demeclocycline) 300 mg–600 mg twice daily. Monitor for renal impairment while the person is taking demeclocycline.

Further reading

Oxford Textbook of Medicine, Vol. 2, pp. 371–372, 1534.

Hypernatraemia

- Symptomatic hypernatraemia can occur with serum sodium above 150 mmol/l.

Causes of hypernatraemia

	Frequently encountered causes	**Less frequently encountered causes**
Cancer	Use of exogenous glucocorticoids causing Cushing's syndrome[‡]	Cushing's syndrome[‡] (ACTH-producing tumours (small cell lung carcinoma with hypokalaemia as the only clue) or CRH-producing tumours such as bronchial carcinoid, pancreatic tumours, thymus tumours)
Other lifelimiting illnesses		Cystic fibrosis*
Intercurrent illnesses	Diuretics*	Lactulose* (osmotic purgative)
	Any person unable to drink normally[†] (especially with decreased level of consciousness)	Renal failure*
		Cushing's syndrome[‡]
		Primary hyperaldosteronism[‡]
		Central diabetes insipidus* (ADH not synthesized or not secreted)

* Water loss greater than salt loss.
[†] Normal total body water content.
[‡] Salt retention greater than water retention.

History
Clues to hypernatraemia include **new onset of fits** with no known cerebral disease, **decreasing level of consciousness**, or **an acute confusional state from cerebral oedema** (p. 28). Review all medications carefully.

Physical examination
Physical examination will often be normal with mild hypernatraemia. Carefully assess hydration including tissue turgor. Examine for tachycardia and hypotension. Signs of significant hypernatraemia include increasing hyper-reflexia, increasing ataxia, and spontaneous muscle twitching. Clues to causes include Cushingoid appearance: fat deposition (face, upper thoracic spine, supraclavicular region, and abdomen) and skin changes (plethora, striae).

Investigations and management
Prognosis measured in hours to days prior to the onset of this problem (symptom control)
Hypernatraemia becomes an incidental finding in the last few hours or days of life. With neurological deficit, it may be reasonable to hydrate gently if hypernatraemia is due to diuretics, lactulose, or renal failure.

Prognosis measured in weeks prior to the onset of this problem (in addition to 'prognosis measured in hours')

Establish the underlying cause. Stop or wean any medications that may be contributing to the problem. Hydrate to euvolaemia in people with total body water deficit. If the cause is dexamethasone or prednisolone, ensure that the person is experiencing the proposed benefit.

Prognosis measured in months to years prior to the onset of this problem (in addition to 'prognosis measured in weeks')

If hypernatraemia is due to ectopic ACTH, successfully treating the underlying malignancy will treat high sodium.

Further reading

Oxford Handbook of Palliative Care, pp. 424–429.

Acute gout

- Gout may manifest as acute joint swelling and pain or as renal disease (calculi or interstitial damage from crystal deposition).

Causes of gout, causes may include…

	Frequently encountered causes	Less frequently encountered causes
Cancer		Following therapy for sensitive tumours (chemo- or radiotherapy)
		Myeloproliferative diseases.
Intercurrent illnesses	Following alcohol intake, surgery, fasting, or major medical illness	Primary gout (mostly under excretion rather than overproduction)
		Psoriasis
		Medications reducing excretion (diuretics, salicylates, cyclosporin)
		Hypertension
		Sarcoidosis
		Hypothyroidism.
		Haemolytic anaemia of any cause
		Secondary polycythaemia

History

For most people with a life-limiting illness, the diagnosis of the first episode of gout will be clear from the **acute painful joint swelling**. The issue is to contrast with chronic gout (tophi usually present), other causes of acute arthritis (mostly symmetrical), and pseudo-gout (propensity for knees).

Physical examination

Examine the joints affected. Check the renal angles for pain (consider renal calculi).

Investigations and management

Prognosis measured in hours to days prior to the onset of this problem (symptom control)

Pain relief relies on NSAIDs either orally or parenterally (ketorolac 10–30 mg SC three times daily).

Prognosis measured in weeks prior to the onset of this problem in addition to 'prognosis measured in hours'

Choices for treating acute episodes of gout include colchicine. An effective dose is likely to cause diarrhoea.

Prognosis measured in months to years prior to the onset of this problem (in addition to the above)

Having treated an acute episode, it will be important to avoid future episodes especially if there is a precipitant such as tumour lysis. If a person has a risk of tumour lysis, actively hydrate before therapy and use allopurinol prophylactically. In people who have had two or more episodes of gout without an obvious precipitant, use allopurinol in the long term.

Further reading

Oxford Textbook of Medicine, Vol. 2, pp. 50–52.

Tumour lysis syndrome

- Tumour lysis is characterized by a rapid rise in serum urate levels (>900 μmol/l) as tumour cells in highly sensitive tumours are lysed soon after chemotherapy or sometimes when radiotherapy is initiated. Occasionally, it may be seen in untreated acute haematological malignancies because of excessive cell turnover.
- Associated biochemical abnormalities include hyperphosphataemia, raised lactate dehydrogenase, and sometimes hypocalcaemia.
- Circulating urate can be deposited widely, including in the distal renal tubules, causing local obstruction and invoking an intense inflammatory reaction.
- Cancers most frequently associated with tumour lysis syndrome include:
  - acute leukaemias
  - high-grade lymphomas
  - small cell lung cancer (less frequently).

Prevention includes aggressive hydration and regular allopurinol (300 mg orally daily) in people with cancers likely to cause the syndrome as chemotherapy is initiated.

Once the syndrome is established, maximally tolerated hydration with normal saline and close monitoring is initiated if the person is not anuric. Renal function should gradually return to normal as uric acid and phosphate levels fall.

Treatment in established renal failure relies on haemodialysis as the renal tubular system becomes clogged with urate crystals or, less commonly, calcium/phosphate compounds.

Further reading

Oxford Textbook of Medicine, Vol. 2, p. 535; Vol. 3, p. 406.

Neurology

☠ Cord compromise

- Spinal cord compression is a medical emergency.
- The diagnosis must be considered in cancer patients with back pain. Investigations and treatment must be initiated as a matter of urgency in order to best preserve function.
- This must be considered in the context of the overall condition and the prognosis of the person.
- Malignant spinal cord compression is the most common cause of cord compromise in people with life-limiting illnesses.
- Clinically, it occurs in 3–5 per cent of cases of people with cancer, with 70 per cent of cases occurring in the thoracic spine, 20 per cent in the lumbosacral spine, and 10 per cent in the cervical spine.
- Back pain without neurological changes is the first presenting symptom in the majority of cases.

Causes of cord compromise

	Frequently encountered causes	**Less frequently encountered causes**
Cancer	Direct extension of vertebral body metastasis	Vertebral body collapse
		Intradural or lepto-meningeal disease
		Tumour extending through the intravertebral foramina
		Vasogenic oedema
		Invasion of the anterior spinal artery by tumour
Intercurrent illness	Cervical disc prolapse	Infection (epidural abscess)
		Haematoma (anticoagulated people)
	Transverse myelitis	Cord infarct
	Multiple sclerosis	Anterior spinal artery occlusion (atrial fibrillation)
	Guillain–Barré syndrome	Vasculitis
		Dissecting aortic aneurysm

History

The most important and common cause of spinal cord compromise is **malignant spinal cord compression**. The need to consider this diagnosis and initiate prompt treatment cannot be overemphasized.

People with spinal cord compression typically present with **back pain**. This pain often pre-dates neurological changes by months. It may be worse on lying flat and may be exacerbated by coughing, bending, or sneezing. The pain may be localized to the back, or people may describe a heavy band-like sensation that radiates anteriorly.

Limb weakness and sensory changes are late changes. The distribution of changes will depend upon the height of the cord involved.

Bladder and bowel disturbance (urinary retention and incontinence, constipation, and faecal incontinence) occur late in the presentation.

Lesions of the cauda equina present with back pain that may radiate down both legs. There may be difficulty in walking because of gluteal muscle weakness. There is loss of perineal sensation. These people will also develop urinary problems (incontinence and retention) and may have faecal incontinence due to loss of anal tone.

Ongoing intrathecal analgesia or a past history of intrathecal analgesia (epidural injections, epidural catheters, intrathecal catheters) raises the possibility of an **epidural or intrathecal abscess**. These people will have fever and complain of severe back pain. Depending upon the level of the problem, they may have other sensory and motor changes as detailed above.

Physical examination

The physical examination findings will differ depending upon the level of cord compromise or may be unremarkable.

There may be tenderness along the bony spine, and a sensory level with pin-prick should be sought. (Light touch, if normal, is not sufficient to exclude a sensory level as it is carried in both posterior columns and spinothalamic tract. Pin-prick is only carried in posterior columns, the area often affected earliest in cord impingement.) Lesions occurring above L1 may initially present with a flaccid paralysis but an upgoing plantar reflex. Later, this will become a spastic paralysis (increased tone, clonus, and increased reflexes) consistent with an upper motor neuron lesion at the level of the lesion and below it.

Physical examination must include an assessment of bladder and bowel function (percuss for a bladder level; rectal examination for anal tone).

A cauda equine lesion will produce lower motor neuron signs. The leg weakness is flaccid and the reflexes are diminished or absent. Examine for a loss of saddle sensation and decreased anal tone. Percuss for a bladder level.

Malignant cord compressions may be multilevel, in which case the physical examination may display mixed signs.

If an intrathecal catheter is *in situ*, check the skin around the injection site for redness, temperature change, or discharge. Palpate for tenderness and check the temperature. Check for signs of meningism.

Investigation and management

Prognosis measured in hours to days prior to the onset of this problem (symptom control)

This is a clinical diagnosis in this group. Further investigations are not indicated.

To maximize comfort, it may still be reasonable to administer **dexamethasone 8 mg SC daily**. This is likely to improve pain control, although other agents (opioids and paracetamol) must be available. **An indwelling catheter** must be inserted and a **bowel regime implemented**. At this stage of life, there may be minimal oral intake. Therefore, daily enemas or suppositories may be sufficient (Microlax enema or Durolax suppository).

In the case of an epidural abscess or infected intrathecal injection site, removal of the catheter depends upon the ongoing effectiveness of the analgesia. Often these devices have been inserted for very difficult pain problems. Despite the local infection, if analgesia is adequate, the device should be left *in situ*. Antibiotics should be administered to help manage the local painful infection. If analgesia has deteriorated, removal of the device and commencement of alternative analgesia is indicated.

Prognosis measured in weeks prior to the onset of this problem (in addition to symptom control)

The challenge again depends upon deciding whether or not people are well enough to tolerate investigations and treatment.

Although the definitive imaging for suspected cord compromise is MRI, in this group **plain X-rays** may be sufficient. Plain X-rays will be positive for vertebral damage in 80 per cent of cases. This is not the case for infection, where more definitive scans will be required (MRI, CT).

These individuals should be commenced on **dexamethasone 8 mg** oral/SC twice daily (morning and mid-day).

A **radiation oncology consultation** must be sought.

A **bowel regimen** must be implemented and bowel actions charted daily. It may be prudent to seek advice from a continence nurse. **An indwelling catheter** may be required.

There may be associated **difficult pain syndromes** due to a combination of somatic and neuropathic pain.

Individuals in whom an infective cause is suspected should undergo imaging if they are well enough. The decision to remove an intrathecal infusion depends upon the adequacy of analgesia. Regardless of whether or not the device is removed, antibiotics should be commenced and drainage of abscesses, if present, under CT guidance should be considered.

Prognosis measured in months to years prior to the onset of this problem (in addition to the above)

The definitive treatment for malignant extradural lesions compressing the cord is usually **radiotherapy** unless the pathology is exquisitely sensitive to chemotherapy (small cell cancer, lymphoma).

An infective cause requires urgent neurosurgical consultation for consideration of drainage.

Where there is vertebral body collapse with bone impingement on the cord, unstable fractures, or areas that have previously had supramaximal doses of radiotherapy, consideration must be given to **urgent surgical decompression**. For most epidural extension of vertebral disease, the lesion is anterior and therefore surgery requires an anterior approach. This is reserved for people who can tolerate the significant catabolic load associated with surgery, which is not well tolerated late in the clinical course of a life-limiting illness.

Cervical lesions may impair diaphragmatic function (C3–5) causing fatal respiratory compromise. This will need to be discussed with the individual and their family as soon as it is recognized.

Pain may be prominent both at the site of bony collapse and radiating from damaged nerves. Adequate paracetamol, opioids, and antineuritics such as amitriptyline should be used early.

Early recognition of reversible cord pathology is crucial. The better the level of neurological function at the time of diagnosis, the more likely it is that neurological function can be maintained.

Further reading

Oxford Textbook of Palliative Medicine, p. 729.

☼ Delirium: acute confusional states

- Delirium is frequently encountered in people with life-limiting illnesses irrespective of the underlying disease.
- Unlike many other clinical settings, a reversible cause for the delirium is found in only 50 per cent of people at the end-of-life.
- Early recognition is the key to minimizing morbidity:
  - **Hyperactive delirium** is typified by drug withdrawal. Unceasing movement and inability to settle are seen late in delirium.
  - **Hypoactive delirium** is typified by encephalopathy, metabolic disorders, or intoxication. Still ask about perceptual disturbances and still test concentration, distractibility, and memory.

Causes of delirium

	Frequently encountered causes	**Less frequently encountered causes**
Metabolic causes	Dehydration	Hyponatraemia
	Hypercalcaemia	Hypernatraemia (mostly due to dehydration)
		Hypoglycaemia
Medications	Anticholinergic load (cumulative—many medications add to anticholinergic load)	Serotonergic syndromes
		Withdrawal (alcohol, benzodiazepines, nicotine)
	Opioids	Glucocorticoids (psychotropic: depression to hypomania)
	NSAIDs	Digoxin
Sepsis	Pneumonia	Spontaneous bacterial peritonitis (with ascites)
	Urinary tract infection	
	Biliary sepsis	
Cerebral pathology	Intracerebral metastases (including miliary disease and leptomeningeal disease)	Encephalitis (primary herpes simplex infections)
		Subdural haematoma (anticoagulants)
		Post-ictal
End-stage organ failure	Renal or hepatic failure (exclude upper GIT bleeding)	Urinary retention
		Constipation

History

Delirium requires four key features for diagnosis:
- disturbance in consciousness that will fluctuate
- change in cognition not explained by pre-existing, established or evolving dementia

- evolution over a short period of time
- evidence that the disturbance is caused by physiological consequences of the general medical condition.

The most accurate history will often be obtained from families and nursing staff. They will often give clear account of the timeframe for the onset of change and its extent.

Physical examination

- These people may be **quiet and withdrawn or agitated and anxious**. Their **speech and train of thought is disordered**. They may be **paranoid** and **hallucinating**.
- Examine to ascertain the cause of the problem. Check **temperature, blood pressure, pulse, and pulse oximetry. Assess hydration**.
- Look for a **source of sepsis** including the chest (pneumonia, bronchitis), skin (cellulitis), spontaneous bacterial peritonitis (if there is ascites), or meningism (photophobia, neck stiffness) (p.48). Look for asterixis.
- Use a **delirium rating scale** which includes current orientation and ability to concentrate.
- Ensure that the physical examination includes an assessment of **urinary output** (percuss for a bladder) and **constipation**.

Investigations and management

Prognosis measured in hours to days prior to the onset of this problem (symptom control)

- **Delirium at the end-of-life requires assessment and management**.
- Review current medications.
- Treatment should be administered whilst assessment is underway. The initial management should be with **haloperidol 0.5–1.0 mg SC** repeated every 20 min until the person is settled.
- In very agitated people, a dose of a **benzodiazepine** may be added (lorazepam 1 mg SL or midazolam 2.5–5.0 mg SC). Delirium should not be treated with benzodiazepines alone or as the initial therapy.
- **Easily reversible aspects of the delirium should be addressed** (e.g. gentle rehydration, treat fever with paracetamol, address pain appropriately, IDC insertion, low-flow oxygen).
- If individuals do not settle with haloperidol and benzodiazepines, **alternative antipsychotics** include levomepromazine (start with 12.5–25 mg via SC infusion); or chlorpromazine 25–50 mg IM immediately and repeat twice or three times daily or olanzepine 2.5–5.0 mg SL daily. Doses must be titrated depending upon the response.

Prognosis measured in weeks prior to the onset of this problem (in addition to symptom control)

- Investigations should be directed to excluding easily treatable causes.
- Check **urea**, **creatinine** (calculate **creatinine clearance** (p.260)), and electrolytes (**hyponatraemia** and **hypercalcaemia** (corrected for albumin (Appendix 5)).
- Check **urea-to-creatinine ratio** (high in upper GIT bleeding, dehydration, use of dexamethasone).

- With evidence of cerebral irritation, do a **cerebral CT**.
- If there is any evidence of sepsis, collect **blood cultures** and **MSU** and organize a **CXR**.
- Check **FBC** for neutrophilia or lymphopenia.
- **At the same time as investigations are being attended to, management should be commenced.**
- Ensure that the person is not able to harm themselves or others. Move to a quiet well-lit environment with aid to assist orientation.
- There must be close observation and reassessment of the delirium every hour until the person is settled and then every 2 hs whilst the person is awake.
- Remember that antipsychotic medications may lead to hypotension and extrapyramidal side-effects, especially in the elderly, increasing the risk of falls.
- If alcohol withdrawal is considered, ensure that thiamine 100 mg IM is administered immediately. These people are best managed with valium 2–5 mg three times daily and adequate hydration. They should be commenced on an alcohol withdrawal chart, and specialist drug and alcohol support should be sought.

Prognosis measured in months to years prior to the onset of this problem (in addition to the above)

- Delirium may take several days longer to clear than the process of normalizing the underlying cause.
- Delirium in the elderly is an independent risk factor for poorer prognosis.

Further reading

Oxford Textbook of Palliative Medicine, pp. 708–713.

☠ Seizures

- Seizures are feared by people at the end-of-life because they are associated with:
  - loss of control
  - loss of dignity
  - unpredictability.

Causes of seizures

	Frequently encountered causes	**Less frequently encountered causes**
Cancer	Primary or secondary lesions (small cell lung, melanoma, and breast) of the CNS	Secondary bleed into a cerebral metastasis
	More frequent in frontal lobe tumours	
End-stage organ failure	Hepatic encephalopathy	Multiple sclerosis
		Secondary fitting with prolonged hypoxaemia in cardiac arrhythmias
Intercurrent illnesses	Pre-existing epilepsy (especially with changed medication metabolism)	Hypoglycaemia
		Meningitis
	Alcohol use	Primary herpes simplex encephalitis
	Drug withdrawal (including benzodiazepines)	

History
History from the person and someone who has observed the episode is invaluable. Sometimes the precipitant may not be identified. The history may help to define the type of seizure.

- Primary generalized seizures are associated with loss of consciousness as they start. Seizures with evidence of signs that cross the midline of the brain are associated with loss of consciousness. Generalized seizures include absences where there is no loss of posture but loss of activity.
- Focal seizures that generalize are rarely associated with early loss of consciousness.
- Partial seizures are focal and may be considered as simple (consciousness maintained) or complex (consciousness impaired). They often have a warning or 'aura'.
- Status epilepticus is a seizure that lasts longer than 30 min or a series of seizures where the person continues to have impaired consciousness from the post-ictal state before the next seizure begins. Differential diagnosis includes vasovagal syncope, which usually has warning with sweating and weakness, and is not associated with post-collapse

confusion unless there is secondary fitting. Cardiac arrhythmias including Stokes–Adams attacks, and ventricular arrhythmias can cause syncope with subsequent fitting, especially if the person cannot fall to a prone position.

Physical examination
- **Physical findings may well be absent**.
- The period of time for which people have a depressed level of consciousness or confusion will vary widely after generalized seizures.
- **Todd's paresis** refers to transient paralysis following seizure activity.

Investigations and management
Prognosis measured in hours to days prior to the onset of this problem (symptom control)
Seizures may be seen in the terminal stages of a life-limiting illness.
The initial intervention is to arrest the seizure. Medications that may be used include:
- diazepam 10 mg IV or rectally (use a mixing tube)
- midazolam 5 mg SC/SL/IV.
The person should then be commenced on definitive antiseizure treatment.
At the end-of-life, appropriate medications include:
- clonazepam (0.5–1.0 mg SL/SC twice daily or 2–4 mg via SC infusion over 24 hs)
- midazolam (20 mg via SC infusion over 24 hs).
In difficult cases when sedation is required phenobarbital (100 mg SC immediately and then 200 mg via SC infusion daily).

Prognosis measured in weeks prior to the onset of this problem (in addition to symptom control)
Check **FBC** (infection), **EUC** (hyponatraemia, electrolyte disturbance, uraemia), **LFT** (liver failure), and **BSL** (hypoglycaemia).

If the person has previously been known to have epilepsy, **check anticonvulsant levels**. If these are subtherapeutic, consider medication interactions, malabsorption, and poor compliance as causes.

A **cerebral CT** with contrast should be performed in the setting of concerns for structural lesions. **MRI** should be limited to people who do not have known cerebral disease or who have an unremarkable CT and continued fitting. **EEG** may be helpful in a small number of people at the end-of-life with fits which are difficult to characterize.

Therapy is directed to reducing the risk of further fitting. If people are able to swallow consider the following treatment options.
- For **focal seizures**, the drugs of choice include sodium valproate (initially 600 mg daily and titrate to response) and carbamazepine (initially 200 mg daily in divided doses and titrate to response).
- For **generalized seizures**, the first drugs of choice include sodium valproate (initially 600 mg daily and titrate) or phenytoin (initially 4–5 mg/kg/day and titrate up to 300 mg as a starting dose).
- In the presence of **cerebral oedema** from malignancy, glucocorticoids should be used initially.

If individuals are unable to swallow:
- phenytoin may be administered by IV injection. Administer a loading dose of 15 mg/kg by slow injection and then commence 300 mg at night.

If seizures are difficult to control:
- phenobarbital may be administered via the SC route. Start with a loading dose of 100 mg immediately and then administer 100–200 mg in divided doses over 24 hs.

Status epilepticus is an emergency. The airway must be protected by positioning. Consider an oral airway or even intubation. Administer oxygen. Establish an intravenous line. The first medications are to try and arrest the seizure. Administer diazepam 2–10 mg IV (or lorazepam 1–2 mg or midazolam 2.5–5.0 mg). After this, commence phenytoin (with a loading dose parenterally of 15 mg/kg by slow IV injection). These medications must not be administered via the same intravenous line as they do not mix.
- check **FBC, EUC, BSL, electrolytes**
- administer **100 mg thiamine IV**
- give **50 ml of 50 per cent dextrose if low BSL, but thiamine must always be given first**

An intensive care consultation should be sought if fitting fails to settle.

Prognosis measured in months to years prior to the onset of this problem (in addition to the above)

New-onset seizures in adults are symptomatic of an underlying problem. Investigations include:
- lumbar puncture if there is concern that there may be cryptococcal meningitis
- cerebral CT scan.

If more than one seizure has occurred, antiseizure medication will be required.

Further reading

Oxford Textbook of Palliative Medicine, pp. 706, 860.

☠ **Meningitis**

Causes of meningitis at the end-of-life

	Frequently encountered causes	**Less frequently encountered causes**
Cancer	Acute myeloid leukaemia (Listeria)	Lymphoma/acute lymphocytic leukaemia (non-infectious lymphocytic)
	Myeloma/lymphoma (Streptococcus pneumoniae)	Meningitis associated with devices (especially VP shunts)
	Carcinomatous meningitis (breast or lung cancer)	Chemical meningitis (intrathecal medications, contaminants)
HIV/AIDS	Cryptococcal meningitis	
	Toxoplasmosis	
End-stage organ failure		Alcoholism (Streptococcus pneumoniae)
		Multiple sclerosis (non-infectious lymphocytic)
		Nephrotic syndrome (hypogammaglobulinaemia with Streptooccus pneumoniae)
		Connective tissue diseases (sarcoidosis, SLE, Behcet's syndrome)
Intercurrent illnesses	Bacteraemia especially urinary tract sepsis (Escherichia coli)	Previous splenectomy (Streptococcus pneumoniae)
	Prolonged immuno-supression from glucocorticoids (Listeria monocytogenes)	Sentinel bleed of arteriovenous malformation
		Medications (NSAIDs, trimethoprim)
		Post-spinal anaesthesia
Community-acquired illnesses	Bacterial meningitis (meningococcal, pneumococcal, crytococcus, TB)	
	Viral (herpes simplex, herpes zoster, Coxsackie, mumps, measles)	

History

Infectious meningitis may have a **short history of headache, irritability, photophobia, and nausea and vomiting**. The person may not be able to describe these changes and a history from family or care-givers must be sought. There is a need to exclude secondary bacterial meningitis in people with an established focus of sepsis.

Early symptoms are vague: malaise, myalgias, and influenza-like changes, followed later by headache and vomiting. Photophobia and drowsiness are late signs.

People with meningeal carcinomatosis may describe severe headaches. These typically occur insidiously over weeks together with neurological deficits that cannot be attributed to a single lesion. These people often have associated intractable nausea or unheralded vomiting (p. 44), lethargy and drowsiness, diplopia, seizures, and pain (neck, back, radicular distribution).

Physical examination

- Check for **vital signs** (blood pressure, pulse, and temperature) as evidence of sepsis.
- People with infective meningitis may be **febrile, bradycardic, and hypertensive with irregular respiration**.
- Check for **Kernig's sign** (pain and resistance with passive knee extension when the hips are flexed) and Brudzinski's sign (hips flex when the head is tilted forward).
- The **level of consciousness may be reduced** and the person may be **irritable**.
- A transient petechial rash may be seen in meningococcal meningitis (shins, forearms, conjunctiva).
- **Classic signs of neck stiffness, photophobia, and fever may not be present in chronic meningitis or severely immunocompromised people**.
- People with meningeal carcinomatosis, often have cranial nerve lesions (cranial nerves III, IV, VI most commonly affected).
- Other physical findings commonly include localized back and neck pain, limb weakness (lower > upper), and dermatomal sensory changes. Neck stiffness is not a routine clinical finding. Raised intracranial pressure is common, and extensor plantar responses are frequently seen.

Investigations and management

Prognosis measured in hours to days prior to the onset of this problem (symptom control)

- **This is a clinical diagnosis. Further investigations are not indicated**.
- Treatment of symptoms must be attended to.
- Presumed infectious causes of meningitis require **treatment of fever** (paracetamol, NSAIDs, control of ambient temperature).
- **Manage headache and other sites of pain** with parenteral analgesia (morphine, hydromorphone). Adjuvant analgesia to address associated neuropathic pain may be indicated.
- These people are often **confused and cerebrally irritated**. They are best managed in a quiet environment. Gentle sedation may be required.
- **Pay attention to continence**. People may be incontinent or have impaired bladder and bowel function due to neurological impairment and associated confusion. An indwelling catheter and a bowel regime may be required.

Prognosis measured in weeks prior to the onset of this problem (in addition to symptom control)

Where an infective cause is expected, **examination of the cerebrospinal fluid is needed urgently**. **Lumbar puncture** may show increased opening pressure (>200 mmH$_2$O), reduced glucose, and lymphocytosis (>4 mm^3). Any polymorph in CSF is abnormal. Raised protein is likely (but can also be seen in multiple sclerosis or Guillain–Barré syndrome without infection). At the same time take blood for **FBC** and **blood cultures**.

People with infective meningitis in this prognostic group will benefit from antibiotics. Seek the organism's identification and sensitivities. If there is risk of *Staphylotococcus aureus*, cover should be with vancomycin titrated to blood levels until cultures are available. If there is a VP shunt, it is unlikely that sepsis will be cleared without removal.

In meningeal carcinomatosis, a gadolinium-enhanced MRI scan will show diffuse meningeal changes, with foci around nerve roots.

Carcinomatous meningitis carries a poor prognosis with limited interventions available to modify the course of the disease. This group may benefit from a trial of dexamethasone 8–16 mg in the morning. It is unlikely they will achieve any benefit from intrathecal or systemic chemotherapy. Radiotherapy directed to sites of pain may provide some symptom relief.

Regardless of the cause of the meningism, treatment of fever and headache are priorities. In people electing not to have further disease-modifying treatment, the major symptom burden comes from raised intracranial pressure and ensuing unheralded vomiting (p. 44).

Prognosis measured in months to years prior to the onset of this problem (in addition to the above)

If infectious meningitis is suspected, this must be treated as a medical emergency and infectious diseases consultation must be obtained immediately.

Simultaneous investigations and treatments must be initiated.

• Ensure **IV access** and treat for shock if systolic BP <80 mmHg.
• Collect blood immediately for **FBC**, **blood glucose**, and **blood cultures**.
• If there is suspicion of meningococcal meningitis, treat immediately with benzylpenicillin 1.2 g.
• If **CT scans** are readily available, organize an urgent head CT and if there is no evidence of raised intracranial pressure, collect **CSF for urgent assessment**. If CT is not readily available, examine for **papilloedema and proceed to lumbar puncture**.
• **Ensure headache and nausea are addressed** with appropriate medications
• Once the blood cultures and CSF are collected, it is appropriate to initiate antibiotics. The choice depends upon the clinical scenario and this is best discussed with an infectious diseases specialist.
  It is worth considering the following:
  • community-acquired meningitis in adults and the elderly may be due to meningococcus or pneumococcus.

- consider herpes simplex encephalitis and treat actively to avoid long-term neurological complications for the person
- immunosuppressed people are additionally at risk of cryptococcal meningitis, listeria, TB, Gram-negative organisms, and *Cryptococcus*
- hospital acquired or post-surgical meningitis may be due to *Klebsiella, Pseudomonas*, or *Staphylococcus aureus*.

People with a presumed diagnosis of malignant meningeal infiltration require dexamethasone 8–16 mg daily. Other symptoms of pain, nausea and vomiting must be addressed.

The prognosis for people with malignant meningeal infiltration is approximately 2–6 months. However, it is important to consult medical and radiation oncology teams, as appropriate interventions may arrest the development of further neurological deficits.

☢ Intracranial bleeding

- This encompasses intracerebral, subdural, and subarachnoid bleeding.
- Any change in level of cognitive function should raise the differential diagnosis of silent intracranial bleeding.

Causes of intracranial pathology

	Frequently encountered causes	Less frequently encountered causes
Subdural haematoma	Epilepsy	Haemodialysis
	Alcohol misuse, anticoagulant therapy	
	The elderly	
Subarachnoid haemorrhage	Acquired aneurysms (age the major risk factor)	
Intracerebral bleeding	Hypertension	Haemorrhage into a cerebral metastasis
	Arteriovenous malformations (age <45)	Haemorrhage into a completed CVA
	Amyloid deposits	Haemorrhage complicating septic emboli (infective endocarditis p. 104)

History

In subdural haemorrhage, only 50 per cent of people can identify head trauma to account for the problem. Fluctuating consciousness occurs late in the clinical course. The majority of people present with headache or vomiting.

Subarachnoid haemorrhage leads acutely to cerebral vasospasm and systemic hypertension. Without trauma, these are almost always due to (acquired) aneurysmal bleeds. Sudden onset of severe headache or loss of consciousness account for most clinical presentations.

Intracerebral haemorrhage is characterized by progressive changes over a short time period. Vomiting and headache are the predominant symptoms. Changes in consciousness are prominent as the bleed progresses.

Physical examination

A person with a subdural haemorrhage is likely to have non-specific signs of cerebral irritation (personality change, irritability, sleepiness, unsteady gait). There may be fluctuation in cognitive function. In some cases, the physical examination may be normal. In other people, there may be focal neurological signs (unequal pupils, hemiplegia). The presentation can mimic delirium.

For subarachnoid bleeding, neck stiffness takes hours to develop and its absence does not exclude subarachnoid blood. Other changes include drowsiness, coma, and focal neurological signs. If focal signs occur early after the onset of the headache, consider cerebral haematoma. If this occurs later, cerebral ischaemia is likely.

Intracerebral bleeds are usually associated with hypertension. Examine for cardiomegaly and fundal changes of hypertension.

Investigations and management

Prognosis measured in hours to days prior to the onset of this problem (symptom control)

These people require **pain relief with opioids and paracetamol**. If the person is clinically dehydrated, start very gentle hydration (0.9 percent NaCl 1 l SC over 24 hs). Changes which suggest a substantial bleed include hypertension and a stiff neck. **Stop anticoagulation. Consider treatment of hypertension** with topical nitrates (glyceryl trinitrate patch 25 mg).

Prognosis measured in weeks prior to the onset of this problem (in addition to symptom control)

- The initial investigation is a **cerebral CT**.
- Whilst awaiting the scan, ensure **IV access and check FBC, EUC, and coagulation studies**.
- If a bleed is suspected, **stop anticoagulation, ensure adequate hydration, and commence symptom control** (analgesia, antiemetics). If the person is very agitated, consider sedation.
- If the underlying aetiology on CT scan is a **subarachnoid haemorrhage**, management includes:
  - **analgesia**
  - **careful hydration** (underhydration may worsen vasospasm)
  - **sedation** if very agitated
  - **cautious control of hypertension** (use calcium-channel blockers to prevent vasospasm).

There is a high risk of further bleeding leading to death.

This contrasts with a subdural haematoma as surgical burr holes may lead to a complete recovery.

- **A bleed into cerebral metastases requires**:
  - **a trial of dexamethasone** (8–16 mg in the morning)
  - **control of headaches**
  - **control of nausea and vomiting**.

Remember that although a bleed into a metastasis is a very serious proposition, this group may improve. Families and carers need to be informed of both the possibilities that the person may rapidly deteriorate and die or that they may transiently improve.

Prognosis measured in months to years prior to the onset of this problem (in addition to the above)

Investigations and management must be simultaneously attended to.

- **Seek neurosurgical and neurological opinions promptly.**
- **Ensure IV access.**
- **Elevate the head of the bed to 30°.**
- **Ensure that the person is placed on bed-rest with analgesia and antiemetics prescribed.**

- Cautiously **manage hypertension and maintain euvolaemia** (to avoid vasospasm).
- If the **head CT is normal and a subarachnoid haemorrhage is suspected, organize a lumbar puncture** (early after the bleed, the CSF is blood-stained; later, xanthochromia develops).

A neurosurgical opinion should be sought following a subarachnoid haemorrhage as surgery is aimed at preventing rebleeds. If the bleed was due to an AV malformation, careful consideration will need to be given to best treatment options in consultation with the neurosurgical unit—surgery, stereotactic radiotherapy, or 'coiling'. (Ten per cent of people rebleed within hours of their initial bleed.)

☠ Raised intracranial pressure

- Any increase in the volume of contents in the fixed space of the cranial vault can lead to intracranial hypertension.
- This occurs because of:
  - increased capillary permeability (tumours, trauma, infection, ischaemia)
  - hypoxic cell death
  - obstructive hydrocephalus.
- Signs and symptoms occur when compensatory mechanisms are overwhelmed.
- The ultimate consequence is decreased cerebral perfusion.

Causes of raised intracranial pressure

	Frequently encountered causes	Less frequently encountered causes
Cancer	Any cerebral tumours	Non-communicating hydrocephalus secondary to tumour or oedema
Intercurrent illnesses	Haemorrhage Intracranial haematomas Ischaemic injury to brain Cerebral abscesses	Medications (tetracycline, oral contraceptive, glucocorticoids, vitamin A, perhexiline) Stage IV hepatic encephalopathy

History

- People with **raised intracranial pressure will complain of headache**. This may be worse on waking from sleep, coughing, and straining. However, headache may not be a prominent symptom and can be absent at times even with significant intracranial hypertension.
- A full **spectrum of altered consciousness can be seen**, ranging from mild irritation to profound obtundation.
- People may complain of **visual disturbances**.
- Additionally, people may describe **nausea and vomiting**. This is often worse in the morning and may settle later in the day.
- A recent history of trauma should be sought.

Physical examination

Check whether the person has **papilloedema** (even this is not always apparent in people with raised intracranial pressure). Check for **multiple cranial nerve** lesions. When there is herniation of the temporal lobe, an ipsilateral lesion of cranial nerve III combined with contralateral body weakness may occur. Bradycardia and hypertension may be present.

Eventually **Cheyne–Stokes** respiration may be present. Later, there may be **decerebrate posturing**.

Investigations and management

Prognosis measured in hours to days (symptom control)

- **Headache and impaired consciousness** are the major problems with raised intracranial pressures.
- Titrate opioids to relieve pain.
- **Unheralded vomiting** can be very troublesome (p. 44). Use metoclopramide 10 mg SC every 8 hs. Consider the addition of haloperidol 0.5–1–5 mg SC at night if nausea is difficult to settle.
- **Dexamethasone** 4 mg SC may reduce both the headache and the nausea and vomiting if the cerebral oedema is due to a tumour.

Prognosis measured in weeks prior to the onset of this problem (in addition to symptom control)

Urgent **cerebral CT** is used to define any underlying pathology. Whilst awaiting the scans:

- insert an **IV cannula**
- collect blood for **FBC, Coags, EUC, LFT, and BSL**
- elevate the head of the bed to 30°
- ensure that **analgesia and antiemetics** are available.

A person with focal neurosurgical signs secondary to a subdural haematoma may benefit from burr holes. Additionally, ensure blood pressure control. Maintain oxygen saturation and correct hyponatraemia. Do not overhydrate (no more than 1000 ml intake in 24 hs).

In people with cerebral oedema secondary to tumours (primary or secondary) it is probably not appropriate to consider radiotherapy as the life expectancy is such that thay are unlikely to derive benifit.

Prognosis measured in months to years prior to the onset of this problem (in addition to the above)

Seek neurosurgical and neurological opinions early. **The initial interventions are to ensure that the person can protect their airway and ensure IV access.**

Cerebral CT is used to define any underlying pathology and may demonstrate compression of the lateral ventricles. **Lumbar puncture** is contraindicated if there is significant oedema on CT scanning as transtentorial herniation can occur.

Given that changes of intracranial hypertension occur in a closed space, a small reduction in intracranial pressure can lead to a substantial improvement in function. Measures that may assist with this include:

- correction of low serum sodium
- maintaining normal blood oxygen and carbon dioxide levels
- consider 200 ml of 20 per cent mannitol over 15–30 min.

Urgent neurosurgical consultation is required if there is tumour, haematoma, or non-communicating hydrocephalus causing the raised intracranial pressure. If a tumour is present commence the person on regular dexamethasone 16 mg in the morning. Carefully monitor Glasgow coma scores (Appendix 6).

If left untreated, raised intracranial pressure carries a very poor prognosis.

Orthopaedic disorders

☼ Vertebral Fracture

- Only one in three vertebral fractures come to medical attention.
- Regardless of the aetiology, the occurrence of one vertebral fracture increases the likelihood of further problems within 12 months.
- Vertebral fractures are most likely to occur in the thoracic and lumbar spine.

Causes of vertebral fractures

	Frequently encountered causes	**Less frequently encountered causes**
Cancer	Bony metastases	
Intercurrent illness	Primary osteoporosis	Hypogonadism
	Osteoporosis secondary to glucocorticoids	Hypothyroidism
		Vitamin D deficiency
		Alcohol

History

- People with vertebral fractures commonly present with **acute onset of back pain that may radiate** anteriorly.
- They may also develop an **acute loss of height** or an **exaggeration of spinal curvature**.
- Rarely, thoracic vertebral fractures may present with acute shortness of breath or neurological symptoms consistent with **spinal cord compression** (p. 204) or **cauda equina compression** (p. 205).

Physical examination

Physical examination may be unremarkable, even in the presence of early cord compromise. There may be **percussion tenderness** at the level of the fracture.

Investigations and management

Prognosis measured in hours to days prior to the onset of this problem (symptom control)

This is a clinical diagnosis and no further investigations are indicated.
Vertebral fractures may be very painful, especially on movement. Adequate analgesia is imperative. This may require the use of opioids (morphine 2.5–5.0 mg SC every 4 hs) and paracetamol (1 g orally/IV or 500 mg rectally four times daily). An anti-inflammatory agent, either steroidal (dexamethasone 4–8 mg SC daily) or non-steroidal (ketorolac 10 mg SC four times daily, indomethacin 100 mg rectally daily) may be of assistance in managing movement-related pain.

Prognosis measured in weeks prior to the onset of this problem (in addition to symptom control)

Plain X-rays of the spine are diagnostic. Depending upon the overall condition of the person, further investigations may be indicated. These include inflammatory markers (ESR, CRP), calcium, alkaline phosphatase, and thyroid function.

Additional analgesia may be achieved by the addition of a single infusion of bisphosphonates (pamidronate 60–90 mg IV, zeledronate 4 mg IV).

Prognosis measured in months to years prior to the onset of this problem (in addition to the above)

In people with unexplained fractures, consideration must be given to an underlying malignancy. An **MRI** is indicated in these people, or in people with a known malignancy.

The most important symptom is **pain**. Vertebral fractures may be very painful and have a major impact on an individual's quality of life. Pain must be addressed promptly to allow people to be as well and as mobile as possible.

Consider **vertebroplasty** in this population but ensure adequate analgesia in the 48 hs immediately after the procedure. **Intercostal nerve blocks** may also be considered in people who fail to achieve analgesia by simple means or who are developing adverse effects from prescribed analgesia for thoracic vertebral collapse.

People with vertebral fractures due to malignancy should be considered for a **trial of dexamethasone** (4–8 mg orally/SC daily) and **radiotherapy**.

The **long-term sequelae from vertebral fractures relate to changes in posture**. With progressive kyphosis, changes to gait can occur, making review by a physiotherapist and consideration of walking aids essential.

The role of calcium and vitamin D supplementation is unclear in verterbral fractures. However, ongoing bisphosphonates have a role in preventing further damage and may assist with pain management.

People with vertebral fractures have an overall increased mortality, with 16 per cent reduction in estimated 5 year survival. Part of the reason for this is the association of vertebral fractures with malignancy.

☢ Threatened or actual fracture of long bones

- Pathological long-bone fractures most commonly occur in the humerus and femur.
- The most common presenting problem for both actual and threatened fractures is pain.
- The detection of impending fractures allows planned interventions to maintain mobility, improve analgesia, and avoid neurological compromise.
- Surgical management of actual and impending fractures should be considered in people with a life expectancy of more than 1 month.

Causes of actual or impending pathological fractures

	Frequently encountered causes	**Less frequently encountered causes**
Cancer	Lytic (breast, non-small cell lung cancer) Sclerotic (prostate)	Sarcoma
Intercurrent illness	Paget's disease of bone Osteoporosis	Metabolic bone disease

History

People with **threatened fractures will present with pain**. Initially, this may be pain on movement which settles with rest. Once a fracture has occurred, there will be a **sudden increase in pain** that may become constant. This is often the only clue to the underlying problem. There is rarely a history of trauma.

Physical examination

There may be very little to find on physical examination of people with impending fractures or there may be localized bone tenderness over the affected region. Once a facture has occurred, there may be **swelling** or **deformity** over the affected bone. **Examination must include an assessment of the neurovascular state of the limb distally**.

Investigations and management

Prognosis measured in hours to days prior to the onset of this problem (symptom control)

This is a clinical diagnosis and investigations are not indicated. If it appears from the clinical examination that a fracture has occurred, it is good symptom control to immobilize the limb to maximize pain relief, in addition to administration of opioids (morphine 2.5–5.0 mg SC every 4 hs in the opioid naive or titrate to analgesia in people already receiving opioids), paracetamol (1 g orally/IV times daily or 500 mg rectally daily), and anti-inflammatory agents (ketorolac 10 mg SC four times daily, indomethacin 100 mg rectally daily).

Despite the very limited prognosis, it may be very good palliation to consider intervention pain relief with an epidural or peripheral nerve block which will allow the person to be comfortably nursed.

Prognosis measured in weeks prior to the onset of this problem (in addition to symptom control)

The most important investigation is a **plain X-ray**. The X-ray must include the joints above and below the long bone in question and be compared with the contralateral side.

Impending fractures are diagnosed by a combination of X-ray changes where lesions occupy more than two-thirds of the bone's cortex and pain sufficient to interfere with function. Hairline pathological fractures may not be visible on plain X-rays and may be better visualized with a CT scan.

An **orthopaedic consultation** should be sought to establish whether or not surgical stabilization is possible. A **radiotherapy consultion** should also be sought in people with malignancy, even those who are not well enough for surgery.

All these people require good pain relief. A regular bisphosphonate may provide additional pain relief if the fracture is due to a malignancy or osteoporosis.

Once a fracture has occurred, **immobilization of the area will improve analgesia**. If people are not well enough for surgery, consideration of splinting the limb (or traction for femoral fractures) must be discussed with the orthopaedic team and physiotherapists.

Prognosis measured in months to years prior to the onset of this problem (in addition to the above)

- These people require **plain X-rays** and an orthopaedic consultation. They may need a **CT scan** to exclude a hairline fracture.
- Check **FBC, EUC, LFT, coagulation studies, TFT, and Ca²⁺**.
- Ensure that these individuals have a **CXR and ECG** in preparation for surgery.
- **Commence DVT prophylaxis**.

The prognosis associated with actual or threatened fracture depends to some extent on the prognosis of the underlying disorder, the site of the problem, and the condition of the surrounding bone. People for whom an operation is not feasible because of advanced disease or comorbidities have a very poor prognosis. People with operable fractures may maintain a prognosis consistent with their disease generally.

Ensure that post-surgery radiotherapy is organized if this condition is secondary to malignancy.

Further reading

Oxford Textbook of Palliative Medicine, pp. 268–271.

☢ Fat embolism syndrome

- The fat embolism syndrome occurs when people become symptomatic because of fat droplets entering the vasculature.
- This typically occurs about 12 hs after an insult such as a bone fracture.
- There may be a range of presentations from mild hypoxaemia to life-threatening respiratory failure.

Causes of fat embolism syndrome

	Frequently encountered causes	**Less frequently encountered causes**
Cancer	Pathological fracture of a long bone	
Intercurrent illness	Traumatic fracture of a long bone	Thrombolysis
	Orthopaedic procedures, surgery	Sickle cell crisis

History

- These people may be very sick.
- They may have **increasing shortness of breath** and may develop respiratory failure. In association with breathlessness they may have fever.
- Neurological manifestations include **drowsiness, confusion, hemiplegia, seizures, and coma**.

Physical examination

- These people are **breathless and hypoxic**. They may be **febrile, tachycardic, and hypotensive**.
- Examine for a **petechial rash**, which typically appears over the oral mucosa and skin of the neck and axilla.
- Neurological examination is remarkable for a **delirium** (p. 28).
- Examine all limbs to ensure that there is no hemiplegia.

Investigations and management

Prognosis measured in hours to days prior to the onset of this problem (symptom control)

- **This is likely to be a terminal event in these people**.
- They require **analgesia, administration of low-flow oxygen, treatment of delirium, and control of bleeding diathesis if present**.
- Ensure that **crisis medications** (p. 52) are available in case there is torrential bleeding.
- If a fracture is present, **immediate stabilization may prevent further fat extravasation and improve comfort**.

Prognosis measured in weeks prior to the onset of this problem
(in addition to symptom control)
- Check **FBC**, **EUC**, **albumin**, and **Ca^{2+}**.
- FBC may show anaemia and thrombocytopaenia. Other investigations may show hypoalbuminaemia and hypocalcaemia. **Fat globules may be visible in the serum and urine**.
- Check **pulse oximetry** and **arterial blood gases** for hypoxaemia. Organize a **CXR** (patchy infiltrate).
- **The management of this problem is supportive**.
- These people may be shocked and will require **fluid resuscitation**. Regular pulse oximetry must be instituted and **oxygen** administered to maintain PaO$_2$ >90 mmHg.
- **Corticosteroids** (methylprednisolone 10 mg/kg/day in divided doses) may improve respiratory function.
- **Attention to symptoms must be considered**. It is likely that these people will be in pain because of the underlying problem. They will be breathless and may have a multifactorial delirium.
- Because of **thrombocytopaenia**, they are at risk of bleeding.

Prognosis measured in months to years prior to the onset of this problem
(in addition to the above)
Acute onset of breathlessness, confusion and petechiae are the hallmarks of this syndrome. These people require **transfer to intensive care for** ventilator support if they have severe respiratory compromise.

If people develop respiratory failure and the adult respiratory distress syndrome, the prognosis is guarded. Without respiratory support, more than 90 per cent of people will suffer respiratory arrest; with support, approximately 60 per cent mortality is expected. There is still a 50 percent chance that those people who survive will develop progressive pulmonary fibrosis.

Mental health

☠ Suicide assessment

Assessment of risk for suicide is the responsibility of every health professional in contact with people who may be perceived to be in difficult circumstances. It includes the assessment of people with a life-limiting illness and their care-givers. Urgently seek early psychiatric assessment in someone who is suicidal.

Suicide risk assessment is complex, and even with good risk assessment people may still commit suicide.

Assess key risk factors including:
- male (16–25, 55–70)
- depression (or other psychiatric disorders)
- low self-esteem
- feelings of excessive guilt
- a fear of being a burden to others
- social isolation
- alcohol and drug use
- physical illness
- feelings of helplessness or hopelessness
- prior suicide attempts
- advancing disease
- uncontrolled symptoms
- acute confusional state with delusions or hallucinations (p. 28)
- recent bereavement
- family history of suicide.

Consideration needs to be given to the degree of intent where a person has:
- thought about suicide
- identified the means for suicide
- acted to make those means ready for suicide
- attempted to end his/her life.

To manage the threat of suicide, identify:
- whether this person can be managed in an out-patient setting, an in-patient setting on a palliative care ward, or in a specialist psychiatric unit
- the suicidal person's support network. Ensure that, with permission, this network is mobilized to provide real support to the person considering suicide
- any precipitating factors that may have focused thoughts on suicide at this time (especially if there is a reversible component to this)
- any reversible cognitive or psychiatric aspects to the current thoughts about suicide including clinical depression (p. 238) or an acute confusional state (p. 208). (In this case, has the person lost the ability to make informed decisions and are they therefore a greater threat to themselves? Anyone who is acutely suicidal and cognitively impaired needs to be considered for an urgent in-patient psychiatric assessment, on occasions without the suicidal person's permission.)

If a person is to remain in the community and does not appear to be at imminent risks of suicide, contract with the person that they will not seek to kill themselves without initially making contact with someone such as their general practitioner or community nurse.

Further reading

Oxford Textbook of Palliative Medicine, pp. 755–756.
Oxford Handbook of Palliative Care, pp. 440–441.

✛ Depression

- The prevalence of depression in people with a life-limiting illness is no different from its prevalence in the population presenting to general practitioners.
- Depression needs to be distinguished from sadness.
- Depression is underdiagnosed and undertreated in people with a life-limiting illness.

Causes of depression

	Frequently encountered causes	**Less frequently encountered causes**
Cancer		Frontal-lobe tumours. Higher rates in people with carcinoma of the pancreas, lung, and kidney
Intercurrent illnesses	Stroke, especially left anterior frontal lobe Higher rates in people with diabetes mellitus, multiple sclerosis, coronary artery disease	Glucocorticoids may cause severe depression as one of their psychotropic effects Amphetamine withdrawal Antihypertensives (beta-blockers, clonidine, reserpine, methyldopa) Levodopa

History

- **Assessment includes previous episodes of depression and current medications**.
- **Assess specifically for suicidality** (p. 236).
- **Do not rely on somatic symptoms** (anorexia, fatigue, psychomotor retardation, or weight loss) as these physical changes overlap with cachexia in life-limiting illnesses.
- Depressed affect, sleep patterns with early morning insomnia, and loss of pleasure in any aspect of life (anhedonia) are important pointers to depression in this population.

Physical examination

- Physical examination will often be normal.
- Consider signs consistent with frontal-lobe spread of malignancy in people with cancers likely to spread to the CNS.
- Check for concrete thinking and primitive reflexes.

Investigations and management

Prognosis measured in hours to days prior to the onset of this problem (symptom control)

Support is the key in people in the terminal phases of their life-limiting illness. Acknowledge that depression is there.

Prognosis measured in weeks prior to the onset of this problem (in addition to symptom control)

Counselling (stress management, problem solving) or supportive psychotherapy (e.g. cognitive behavioural therapy) is the first aspect in treating mild or moderate depression.

Adjustment disorder with depressed mood is also best treated with supportive interventions rather than antidepressants as first-line therapy.

Major depression needs early identification and treatment with antidepressants. Choice is largely determined by intercurrent illness (SSRIs have less cardiac toxicity) and interactions with existing medications (Ch. 2). Although the onset of action may be as long as 2 months, many people will start to notice benefit within 2 weeks, including improved sleep patterns and lighter affect.

Prognosis measured in months to years prior to the onset of this problem (in addition to above)

In people not responding to an adequate trial (dose and duration) of first-line antidepressants, consider consultation with a psychiatrist.

Further reading

Oxford Textbook of Palliative Medicine, pp. 750–755.
Oxford Handbook of Palliative Care, pp. 424–429.

☼ Hypomania

Between 1 and 2 per cent of the population have evidence of bipolar disorder.

Causes of hypomania

	Frequently encountered causes	**Less frequently encountered causes**
Intercurrent illnesses	Glucocorticoids	Levodopa
		MAOIs
		Sympathomimetics
		Tricyclic antidepressants

History
- **Hypomania may be associated with flight of ideas, motor and verbal overdrive, illusions, grandiose plans, and reduced sleep time.**
- The onset is often abrupt, and of relatively short duration (compared with mania), and may be associated with increases in energy out of proportion to the life-limiting illness.
- **Hypomania needs to be distinguished from an acute confusional state** (p. 28).
- It also needs to be distinguished from frontal-lobe lesions that may cause euphoria or social disinhibition.

Physical examination
Physical examination will often be normal.

Investigations and management
Prognosis measured in hours to days prior to the onset of this problem (symptom control)
In hypomania in the terminal phases of a life-limiting illness use haloperidol 0.5–2.5 mg orally/SC twice daily. Other choices include olanzapine 2.5–10 mg or risperidone 0.5–2 mg orally in divided doses. These doses will need to be titrated to effect.

Prognosis measured in weeks prior to the onset of this problem (in addition to symtom control)
There are two therapeutic aims of intervention:
- **moderating** mood
- **calming** the person acutely.

The first is best achieved with antipsychotics and the second may require the additional use of benzodiazepines such as diazepam 5–20 mg, depending on the person's body habitus and previous exposure to benzodiazepines, repeated every 2 hs until there is a therapeutic effect.

Other medications which may be used to moderate mood include sodium valproate and carbamazepine.

Prognosis measured in months to years prior to the onset
of this problem (in addition to prognosis measured in weeks)

If this is an initial episode of hypomania or part of a pattern of bipolar changes, consider consultation with a psychiatrist if prognosis is measured in months.

Further reading

Oxford Textbook of Medicine, Vol. 3, p. 1393.
Oxford Textbook of Palliative Medicine, p. 863.

Anxiety

- Many people experience anxiety from time to time but this does not meet the criteria of panic or anxiety disorders.
- **Panic attacks** are characterized by a short period with:
  - severe autonomic symptoms (palpitations, sweating or flushes, tremor, light-headedness)
  - somatic symptoms (shortness of breath or choking, chest or abdominal pain)
  - cognitive changes (feeling of dissociation, fear of losing control).
- **Stress management and cognitive behavioural therapy** have important roles when physical causes for the symptoms have been excluded on first presentation.
- In specific circumstances a short course of a benzodiazepine such as oral diazepam 2 mg twice daily may be justified if there are frequent episodes in a short space of time.
- **Panic disorder** is seen where there are recurring panic attacks with no apparent trigger, leading to ongoing concerns for that person or changed behaviour that persists for more than 1 month.
- **Acute stress** can occur after any traumatic event. Some reactions may be distant from the event but reflect the impact of that event. Acute stress reactions should rarely be managed with medications. Debriefing after such an event may be of some benefit.
- **Adjustment disorder with anxious mood** is seen within 3 months of an identified stressor that is not associated with any long-term patterns of behaviour or mental illness. The best treatment is supportive, with counselling, relaxation. stress management, or cognitive behavioural therapy. The aim is to help the person adapt to new circumstances. At times there may be a place for a short (2-week) course of an anxiolytic such as diazepam 2 mg twice daily.
- **Generalized anxiety disorder** is seen in the longer timeframe (>6 months). Symptoms include feeling unsettled, fatigue, poor concentration, irritability, muscle tension, and poor sleep patterns. As this is a chronic problem, it is worthwhile ensuring psychiatric input as management should include oral venlafaxine 75 mg in the morning or oral paroxetine 10 mg in the morning titrated to effect. The effects of these antidepressants are seen to work in people who are not clinically depressed. Tremor and palpitations may be treated with a low-dose beta-blocker such as oral propanolol 10 mg twice daily.

Further reading

Oxford Textbook of Palliative Medicine, pp. 748–750.
Oxford Handbook of Palliative Care, pp. 421–423.

Complex grief

- There is a wide range of physical, emotional, and social responses that fall within the definition of 'normal' grief.
- Even in the palliative care setting, death is still perceived to be unexpected by many care-givers.
- Both the person with the life-limiting illness and their family and friends are likely to experience grief and loss from the time that a life-limiting illness is diagnosed.
- Grief and bereavement is not a linear process of transition. It is a complex process of adjustment which will see people cycle through a large range of feelings and experiences over quite long periods of time.
- Chronic grief is where people are unable to move on with their lives and where the symptoms of grief are unchanged over years.
- Special concern for more complex longer-term grief with more difficulty making the transition to life without the person may be seen under the following circumstances.
  - High levels of interdependence in the relationship with the person who is dying or has died.
  - Identifiable and sustained negative aspects of the relationship (e.g. physical or emotional abuse). Expressing the full range of emotions can be difficult except in a trusted therapeutic relationship. Such a person may present in the acute care setting years after the death of the person concerned with little evidence of re-establishing social networks or social re-integration.
- Death of a child, a young sibling, a spouse, or a partner is a loss that challenges personhood for many people. There are short- and long-term concerns as to how best to support people in this setting. Acutely, support is aimed at allowing expression of grief within the social context of that person,
- Complicated grief is considered when, over long periods of time, grief continues to be associated with:
  - intense emotions
  - prolonged changes in social functioning, work, and other roles
  - disturbed sleep and no evidence of these issues improving over long periods of time.

It is imperative to exclude concomitant psychiatric diagnoses such as generalized anxiety disorder or depression.

Further reading

Oxford Textbook of Palliative Medicine, pp. 1141–1142.
Oxford Handbook of Palliative Care, pp. 749–762.

Endocrine problems

☠ Hypoglycaemia

- Hypoglycaemia is the most common metabolic disorder.
- It is defined as a plasma glucose <2.5 mmol/l.
- Although the problem is clearly defined, the symptom threshold is widely varied.
- Hypoglycaemia needs to be considered in a range of end-stage diseases other than diabetics being treated with insulin or oral hypoglycaemics.
- **The most common cause of hypoglycaemia in known diabetics is insulin and oral hypoglycaemics.**

Causes of hypoglycaemia in non-diabetics

	Frequently encountered causes	Less frequently encountered causes
Cancer	Cancer cachexia	Insulinoma
	Reduced food intake	Paraneoplastic disease
	Liver tumours (primary or metastatic)	Immune hypoglycaemia (Hodgkin's disease)
		Retroperitoneal fibrosarcomas
End-stage organ failure	Liver failure	Septic shock
		Panhypopituitarism
		Addison's disease

History

There are two main classes of symptoms of hypoglycaemia:
- **Autonomic**: tremor, sweating, palpitations, hunger.
- **Neuroglycopaenic**: confusion, altered behaviour, slurred speech, drowsiness, seizures, coma.

These may all be blunted in the elderly, people receiving beta-blocking medications, or individuals receiving sedative medications.

Physical examination

In the setting of any **unexplained neurological deterioration** (drowsy, confused, sweating, agitated, aggressive), check blood glucose levels.

Investigations and management

Prognosis measured in hours to days prior to the onset of this problem (symptom control)

- In a known diabetic who is still receiving glucose-lowering treatment, a finger-prick BSL should be checked.
- If well enough and able to protect their airway, these people should receive oral glucose or dextrose. If they are not able to take oral medications, consider 25 ml of 50 per cent dextrose IV.
- Hypoglycaemia in people with cachexia, extensive liver dysfunction, or replacement of liver with tumour are unlikely to respond to glycogen.

- In the last stage of life, oral hypoglycaemic medications should be discontinued. If insulin dependent, stop long-acting agents. Rapid-onset insulin (e.g. actrapid) should be substituted and blood sugar monitoring should continue. BSL should be kept in a broad range that is less likely to be associated with symptoms (>8 mmol/l and <14 mmol/l).

Prognosis measured in weeks prior to the onset of this problem (in addition to symptom control)

Check **finger-prick BSL and formal BSL**. Do not wait for the results of the formal BSL. Immediate interventions include the following:-
- If unconscious, protect airway.
- If the person can safely swallow, give glucose by mouth.
- If not, administer 50 per cent glucose IV into a large-bore vein with a saline flush. If there is any question of previous long-term alcohol intake, give with thiamine 100 mg to avoid inducing Wernicke's encephalopathy.
- Follow the oral sugar with a carbohydrate load (e.g. bread).
- If the person is a known type 1 diabetic, glucagon 1 mg may be administered IM or IV (avoid SC in an emergency because of unreliable absorption. (In type 2 diabetes mellitus it will stimulate insulin secretion as well as glycogenolysis and so should not be used).

Once the individual has recovered from this acute episode, the glycaemic control needs to be reviewed.

Renegotiating the aims of glycaemic control can be difficult. Liberalize diet. Reduce or withdraw oral hypoglycaemics in type 2 diabetes and reduce doses of long-acting insulin in type 1 diabetics.

Prognosis measured in months to years prior to the onset of this problem (in addition to the above)

It is reasonable to expect that individuals should recover quickly. However, if recovery is prolonged, recheck the BSL and consider the addition of dexamethasone 4 mg IV four times daily. This is to reduce associated cerebral oedema that may accompany a prolonged and severe episode of hypoglycaemia. Once they have recovered, repeat BSL and in all people perform a septic work-up.

If a person is taking a sulphonylurea, check that renal function has not deteriorated. Renal impairment may prolong the hypoglycaemic effects.

In non-diabetics who are hypoglycaemic, check the following:
- C-peptide (insulinoma)
- insulin levels (insulinoma, exogenous insulin, sulphonylurea administration)
- thyroid function (thyrotoxicosis)
- random cortisol levels (pituitary and adrenal failure)
- hepatic function (liver failure, excess alcohol).

Further reading

Oxford Textbook of Palliative medicine vol. 3, p. 717.
Oxford Handbook of Palliative care pp. 374, 376.

:☣: **Hyperglycaemia**

- The most serious hyperglycaemic complications of diabetes are diabetic ketoacidosis (type 1 diabetes) and hyperosmolar hyperglycaemia (type 2 diabetes).
- Hyperglycaemia in non-diabetic people occurs in extremely unwell individuals and may worsen an already poor prognosis because of the risk of impaired fluid balance, impaired immune function and increased inflammation, and increased risk of thrombosis.

Causes of hyperglycaemia in non-diabetics

	Frequently encountered causes	**Less frequently encountered causes**
Cancer	Insulin resistance in pancreatic cancer	
End-stage organ failure		High-glucose peritoneal dialysis fluids
Intercurrent illnesses	Infection Inflammation Excessive intake (TPN, 5 percent dextrose) Corticosteroids	Medications (thiazide diuretics, sympathomimetics, tacrolimus, cyclosporin)

History

In type 1 diabetes, the onset of hyperglycaemia complicated by keto-acidosis is usually short (<24 hs) with precipitants including:

- infection
- acute myocardial infarction
- pancreatitis
- medications (glucocorticoids, thiazide diuretics, sympathomimetics, tacrolimus, cylosporin)
- alcohol binge.

People present with polyuria, polydipsia and polyphagia, nausea and vomiting, abdominal pain, increasing fatigue, and altered consciousness

In type 2 diabetes, the onset of hyperglycaemia complicated by a hyperosmolar state is often very subtle over a period of days. Confusion or drowsiness suggests significant CNS impairment.

In non-diabetics, the person hyperglycaemic may be thirsty and polyuric. It may be an incidental finding on routine biochemical testing.

Physical examination

- **Assess hydration** (tissue turgor, blood pressure, pulse, urine output).
- A **full neurological assessment** is indicated (level of consciousness, cognition).
- **Deep sighing respirations (Kussmaul breathing)** may be present. The person may be either hypothermic or febrile if an infection is the presenting precipitant.

Investigations and management
Prognosis measured in hours to days prior to the onset of this problem (symptom control)
- It is appropriate to **investigate BSL by finger-prick** testing.
- More invasive blood tests are not indicated.
- A **urine specimen may be collected for ketones**.

Despite the limited prognosis of these people, it is still necessary to **reduce the BSL to <14 mmol/l** to minimize the symptoms of polyuria, thirst, nausea and vomiting, and drowsiness. This is best done by using a **gentle sliding-scale insulin regime with short-acting** insulin (human Actrapid, Humulin S).

BSL (mmol/l)	Insulin dose (Actrapid)
<10	No insulin
10.1–15.0	4 U
15.1–20.0	6 U
>20	8 U

Hydration should be considered and fluid gently replaced if necessary (0.9 per cent NaCl either SC or IV at a rate of 1 l/24 hs. Medications that may precipitate the elevated blood sugar level should be ceased if possible.

Prognosis measured in weeks prior to the onset of this problem (in addition to symptom control)
People with diabetic ketoacidosis and hyperosmolar hyperglycaemia are very unwell. The aim should be to reduce symptom burden.

Assess formal **blood glucose level.** Check **serum electrolytes (especially K⁺ and Na⁺** which may be artificially high, and **renal function** which may be grossly impaired), **serum osmolality, arterial blood gases** to assess acid–base status, and **urine for ketones**. Check for any source of **sepsis** (urine analysis, CXR, blood cultures).

Insulin needs to be administered. Initially, it may be appropriate to do this using a sliding-scale regime with BSL, checked every 2 hs. Long-acting insulin (Mixtard) should be commenced later.

Restore adequate hydration and correct electrolyte abnormalities. It is reasonable to repeat the serum electrolytes and renal function tests daily.

People need to be observed for cognitive decline that may suggest cerebral oedema or increasing shortness of breath due to (non-cardiac) pulmonary oedema.

Non-diabetic individuals in this group who develop hyperglycaemia should also have their formal BSL checked. Further investigations include collection of blood for serum electrolytes, renal function tests, and a septic screen. More intensive investigations are not indicated.

Prognosis measured in months to years prior to the onset of this problem (in addition to the above)

Hyperglycaemia presenting in known diabetics requires prompt attention.

In type 1 diabetes, ketoacidosis must be considered in people who present with high blood glucose who are systemically unwell. This is a medical emergency and the following investigations and treatments must be initiated whilst a high dependency consultation is sought:

- serum electrolytes, renal function, HCO_3, amylase, serum osmolality, Mg^{2+}, PO_4
- FBC
- urinalysis for ketones
- septic screen (blood cultures, urinalysis, CXR)
- arterial blood gases
- start IV insulin 10 U (Actrapid) and commence hydration (1 l 0.9 per cent NaCl immediately then 1 litre over the next hour, then 1 l over 2 hs, and continue in this manner based on the individual fluid balance)
- commence an IV insulin infusion (50 U Actrapid in 50 ml 0.9 per cent NaCl), with the infusion rate based on the hourly BSL; check serum electrolytes after 24 hs
- check vital signs hourly
- insert an indwelling catheter and monitor urine output hourly
- commence DVT prophylaxis
- ensure that the decline in BSL is **not** precipitous as this increases the likelihood of cerebral oedema
- treat suspected infection with intravenous antibiotics; do not wait for the results of the septic screen.

Hyperosmolar hyperglycaemia occurs in type 2 diabetics. This is an extremely serious situation which typically occurs in older people. These individuals may present with dehydration and a BSL >35 mmol/l. This is a medical emergency and the following investigations and treatments should be initiated whilst a high dependency consultation is sought.

- serum electrolytes and renal function, serum osmolality
- FBC
- septic screen
- rehydrate with 0.9 per cent NaCl
- repeat BSL every hour whilst rehydration is occurring; it may not be necessary to use an insulin infusion; it is imperative to avoid rapid changes in electrolytes or BSL
- commence DVT prophylaxis.

Hyperglycaemia in hospitalized people who are not diabetics requires attention when BSL >12 mmol/l.

In the medically unstable, the most appropriate management is with regular insulin (e.g. Mixtard 30/70) rather than sliding-scale insulin. It is important to seek specialist endocrine input. These people and any individual who is found to have a random BSL of >6.9 mmol/l in hospital should be tested for diabetes within a month of hospital discharge.

Further reading

Oxford Textbook of Medicine, vol 2, pp.327, 336, 346, 376
Oxford Textbook of Palliative Medicine , 3rd ed, p. 698
Oxford Handbook of Palliative Care, p. 374

☠ Hypoadrenal crisis

- Addisonian or hypoadrenal crisis is a rare event.
- The symptoms and signs are non-specific and may be mistaken for other serious medical problems (e.g. sepsis, haemorrhage, acute abdomen).
- If missed, it may be a fatal event, and so a high index of suspicion is needed in people who are otherwise unwell and have a sudden deterioration in condition.

Causes of hypoadrenal crisis

	Frequently encountered causes	Less frequently encountered causes
Cancer		Bilateral adrenal metastases
		Aminoglutethimide
Intercurrent illnesses	Sudden withdrawal of long-term glucocorticoids	Autoimmune adrenal disease
	Superimposed stressors (e.g. septicaemia) on a background of glucocorticoid use	Bilateral adrenal haemorrhage (especially people on anticoagulants)
		Bilateral adrenal infarcts
		Pituitary apoplexy
		Meningococcal sepsis
		TB
AIDS		Ketoconazole
		AIDS (opportunistic infections)

History

In a full-blown **hypoadrenal crisis, people present with hypotensive shock**. This occurs because of sodium loss with consequent fluid loss, low renin and prostacycline levels, and decreased response to catecholamines.

More non-specific symptoms include **unexplained fever**, abdominal pain mimicking an acute abdomen, **nausea** and **vomiting**, **lethargy**, **dizziness**, **confusion**, **myalgia**, **arthralgia**, and ultimately **coma**.

Physical examination

- **Tachycardia**, **fever**, and **shock** (tissue turgor, blood pressure including postural drop, pulse, urine output).
- Assess level of consciousness (Glasgow coma score (Appendix 5) and higher centres (Mini Mental Status Examination (Appendix 4)).
- Pigmentation and vitiligo only occur in people with chronic adrenal insufficiency.

Investigations and management
Prognosis measured in hours to days prior to the onset of this problem (symptom control)
- People with suspected hypoadrenal crisis who have a previous history of corticosteroid use should receive corticosteroids (hydrocortisone 100 mg IV or dexamethasone 4–8 mg SC) immediately.
- Treat other symptoms of pain, nausea and vomiting, and increasing confusion as necessary.

Prognosis measured in weeks prior to the onset of this problem in addition to prognosis measured in hours to days (in addition to symptom control)
- Check **serum electrolytes**,($\downarrow$ K^+,$\uparrow$ Na^+) **renal function**, and **urinary sodium** levels (abnormal urinary sodium loss, altered renal function secondary to fluid loss).
- If there is a decreased level of consciousness, **check BSL** for hypo- or hyperglycaemia.
- A **full septic work-up** is indicated (FBC, MSU, blood cultures, CXR).
- If the person does not have a past history of corticosteroid use, an **abdominal CT** to image the adrenals is indicated.
- Management of the problem includes the following:
  - **rehydration** with IV fluids
  - **commence hydrocortisone 100 mg IVI** every 6 hs
  - **commence IV broad-spectrum antibiotics** (aminoglycoside, third generation cephalosporin)
  - **monitor for hypoglycaemia**.
- When more stable, the hydrocortisone may be reduced to 50 mg daily and tapered down to 5–10 mg daily. Fludocortisone (starting dose of 0.05 mg daily) is not indicated acutely. It may be necessary if postural hypotension continues.
- It will be necessary to ensure that steroids are continued for the rest of this individual's life.

Prognosis measured in months to years prior to the onset of this problem (in addition to the above)
In people in whom an adrenal crisis is suspected, management and early investigations must be performed simultaneously. An **endocrine consultation should be sought**.
- Take blood for **random cortisol** and **ACTH, BSL, EUC, TFT, septic screen**.
- **Commence rehydration**. Initially a plasma expander may be necessary; then replace with 0.9 per cent NaCl
- Monitor **blood glucose and administer IV 50 per cent glucose if necessary**.
- Once the person is stabilized, the cause of the hypoadrenal episode will need to be investigated further in people who were not previously taking steroids.
- Investigations include an **abdominal CT scan** and Synacthen test.

Further reading
Oxford Textbook of Medicine vol 2, p. 251

☼ **Thyroid storm**

- Acute presentations of hyperthyroidism are characterized as a 'thyroid storm'.
- This is a presentation with a spectrum of non-specific signs and symptoms where the diagnosis will only be made with a high index of suspicion in relevant people.

Causes of a hyperthyroid crisis

	Frequently encountered causes	Less frequently encountered causes
Cancer		Thyroid cancer
End-stage organ failure		Acute myocardial infarct
Intercurrent illnesses	Exposure to an iodine load (radiographic dyes)	Amiodarone
		Sepsis
	Any pre-existing thyroid disease (painful subacute thyroiditis may proceed to thyroid storm after a viral illness)	Omission of thyroid-suppressing medications
		Overmedication on thyroid replacement therapy

History

People present systemically unwell with **fever and tachycardia**. The tachycardia may be associated with arrhythmias including atrial fibrillation and other supraventricular tachycardias.

Additionally, people may be **confused, agitated, or even moribund**.

They may also have GIT symptoms include nausea and vomiting, **diarrhoea, and abdominal pain that may mimic an acute abdomen**.

Physical examination

- Physical examination may reveal **tachycardia, warm skin, tremor**, and **hyper-reflexia**.
- Other physical signs may be largely absent.
- Evidence of lid-lag, proptosis, and goitre should be sought but are rarely found.

Investigations and management

Prognosis measured in hours to days prior to the onset of this problem (symptom control)

- This is a **clinical diagnosis that should be based on past history and the current clinical situation**.
- Agitation, if present, will need to be addressed with antipsychotic medications (chlorpromazine 50 mg IM or orally twice or three times daily, levomepromazine 25–50 mg via SC infusion).

- **Treat tachycardia** with propanolol (40 mg orally three times daily if able to tolerate oral medications or IV 1 mg over 1 min and repeat up to eight times if necessary).
- **Treat fever** with tepid sponging and paracetamol 1 g orally/IV or 500 mg rectally four times daily.
- **Control vomiting and abdominal pain**. Vomiting may be profuse from high gastric outputs.

Prognosis measured in weeks prior to the onset of this problems (in addition to symptom control)

- Despite the limited prognosis of this group, **an endocrine consultation is indicated** as the mortality from this problem is high.
- Thyrotoxicosis may be associated with a significant symptom burden and so directed management is indicated. However, given the overall limited prognosis, transfer to a high dependency unit is not indicated in this group.
- **Check thyroid function** tests.
- **Blood glucose and corrected serum calcium levels** may be raised.
- **Mild renal impairment** may be present.
- A cholestatic picture may be seen with **LFTs**.
- Leukocytosis is frequently seen on FBC.
- If the person is able to swallow, **commence oral carbimazole 15–25 mg** four times daily. Administer via NG tube if necessary.
- **Rehydrate** with 0.9 per cent NaCl.
- Consider antibiotics if there is focal evidence of infection.

Prognosis measured in months to years prior to the onset of this problem (in addition to above)

This is a medical emergency. An urgent endocrine and high dependency consultation must be sought immediately. Whilst this is occurring, the following investigations and management should be implemented.

- Take blood for **T_3, T_4, EUC, LFT, FBC, random cortisol, blood cultures**.
- **Hydrate** with 0.9 per cent NaCl.
- Sedate if very agitated.
- Administer propanolol 1 mg IV over 1 min and repeat as necessary.
- Insert an **NG tube if vomiting** and administer IV antiemetics (prochlorperazine 12.5 mg IV/IM or haloperidol 0.5 mg SC).
- Transfer to a high dependency unit as soon as possible. The acute presentation of thyroid storm carries a mortality rate of 30 per cent.

Further reading

Oxford Textbook of Medicine, vol 2, p 218

Myxoedema coma

- This is mostly a diagnosis in people with known hypothyroidism.

Causes of hypothyroid crisis

	Frequently encountered causes	**Less frequently encountered causes**
Intercurrent illnesses	Non-compliance with thyroid medications	Amiodarone
	Sepsis	Trauma
		Exposure to cold
		Opioids
		Sedatives

History

- This occurs in people who are known to be hypothyroid (surgery, radioactive iodine).
- Precipitants which may lead to acute deterioration that may be sought on history include non-compliance with medications, infection, trauma, or new onset of an additional acute medical problem which may cause physical stress or render the individual unable to take medications.

Physical examination

- The **signs of hypothyroidism may be present** to give a clue: thin hair, dry coarse skin, enlarged tongue, delayed deep tendon reflexes, and pre-tibial oedema.
- Systemically, **bradycardia and hypotension** are likely to be present.
- **Hypothermia and lethargy** are prominent.
- **Slow mentation** which has gradually deteriorated is an important clue.
- Abdominal examination may reveal a **distended abdomen** secondary to decreased gut motility and megacolon.

Investigations and management

Prognosis measured in hours to days prior to the onset of this problem
The most likely scenario at this stage of life is the development of this problem when individuals can no longer swallow their thyroid replacement.

Prognosis is very poor in this clinical setting and these people must be managed in a manner that is focusing on their comfort. They may be hypoxaemic, and low-flow oxygen via nasal prongs is indicated. They may be hypothermic and so warm ambient temperatures and blankets are indicated. Despite the short prognosis, ensure that these people are not dehydrated.

Prognosis measured in weeks prior to the onset of this problem
(in addition to symptom control)
- **Myxoedema coma carries a poor prognosis even with treatment**.
- If there has been an acute deterioration due to an acute and easily reversible cause (sepsis, AMI), further interventions may be appropriate.

- This situation needs to be managed with caution. **Despite the poor prognosis, consult an endocrinologist**.
- Take bloods for **TFT (TSH, T$_4$, T$_3$), EUC, BSL, FBC**, and **blood cultures**.
- Thyroid function will show a high TSH and low T$_4$. Hypoglycaemia and hyponatraemia are frequently seen.
- **Check for any source of sepsis** (urine analysis, CXR, blood cultures, WCC with differential).
- High **serum creatinine kinase levels** and a high mean cell volume on red cell morphology are consistent with the diagnosis.
- Check **oxygen saturation** and commence oxygen if hypoxaemic.
- Treat **hypoglycaemia** if present.
- Commence **hydrocortisone 100 mg IV three times daily or dexamethasone 4 mg SC twice daily**.
- **An intravenous line should be inserted and T$_3$ 5–20 µg administered over 12 hs**. An endocrinologist should review the dose. This dose should be repeated for 3 days. If well enough, oral T$_4$ may be given.
- **Rehydrate very cautiously** as there is a chance of precipitating cardiac failure.
- Ensure that these people are **kept warm**.

Prognosis measured in months to years prior to the onset of this problem (in addition to above)

These people require urgent endocrine and high dependency consultation. The following investigations and interventions should be initiated:
- check **ABG**
- ensure **intravenous access**
- carefully observe for any signs of **cardiac failure**.

A mortality rate of 20 per cent is associated with hypothyroid coma. This situation requires transfer to a high-dependency unit with thyroid hormone replacement supervised by an endocrinologist.

Further reading

Oxford Textbook of Medicine, vol 2, p. 215

ⓘ **Hypercalcaemia**

- The rate of rise of blood calcium levels dictates the symptom presentation. A rapid rise in calcium may lead to a wide spectrum of problems. In contrast, a slow rise may be an incidental diagnosis.
- In malignancy, raised serum calcium may be related to:
  - lytic bone lesions
  - production of parathyroid hormone-related peptide (PTHrP)
  - deregulated conversion of 25-vitamin D to 1,25(OH)$_2$-vitamin D.
- Correction of serum calcium for albumin levels can be calculated in a number of ways. A simple way is
  corrected Ca = serum Ca + [(40−albumin g/l) × 0.02].

Causes of hypercalcaemia

	Frequently encountered causes	**Less frequently encountered causes**
Cancer	Cancers (most commonly breast, lung, myeloma, lymphoma, renal)	
Intercurrent illnesses		Hyperparathyroidism Sarcoid Vitamin D intoxication Immobility Pancreatitis

History

- **Altered mentation is prominent** in rapidly rising calcium, with irritability, drowsiness, lethargy, seizures, or even coma.
- **Anorexia, nausea** and **vomiting** are frequently encountered. People may have polyuria and **polydipsia**.
- **Constipation** and **muscle weakness** may also be present.

Physical examination

- Assess the **degree of dehydration** (tissue turgor, blood pressure, pulse, urine output).
- Cardiovascular assessment needs to include pulse (exclude sinus bradycardia, or second-degree heart block).
- Assess level of consciousness and formally test cognition.
- **Severe constipation** is often present with a distended uncomfortable abdomen. Auscultate for bowel sounds as a paralytic ileus may be present.

Investigations and management

Prognosis measured in hours to days prior to the onset of this problem (symptom control)

- **In very unwell people entering the final hours of life, no interventions to reduce calcium are necessary**.
- No investigations should be performed.
- Those with a prognosis of days may feel more comfortable with **gentle hydration** (NaCl 1 l via SC infusion over 24 hs) combined with SC calcitonin (50–100 IU daily or twice daily). This may allow correction of the hypercalcaemia more rapidly than IV bisphosphonates which may take up to 48 hs or longer to have an effect in the frail elderly.

Prognosis measured in weeks prior to the onset of this problem (in addition to symptom control)

- **Check serum electrolytes and renal function** (pre-renal impairment from nausea and vomiting, polyuria, inability to drink due to somnolence).
- Pancreatitis may be associated with hypercalcaemia; **check amylase**.
- If there is an unlikely association between the life-limiting illness and hypercalcaemia (e.g. prostatic cancer), check parathyroid hormone levels.
- **Commence hydration** with 0.9 per cent NaCl 1 l IV. The aim is to administer 2 l in 24 hs. This will depend upon the fragility of the person.
- **Forced diuresis is not necessary**. Carefully monitor fluid status to avoid precipitating cardiac failure. It is necessary to repeat EUC daily.
- **Administer an IV bisphosphonate** (disodium pamidronate 30–90 mg over 1–2 hs, or clodroante 1.5 g over 4 hs, or zoledronic acid 4 mg over 15 min).
- **In people with haematological malignancies, commence dexamethasone 4–8 mg SC mane**.
- Approximately 20 per cent of people fail to respond to hydration and bisphosphonates. This is a poor prognostic group, with life expectancy measured now in days to weeks.

Prognosis measured in months to years prior to the onset of this problem (in addition to the above)

- If this was the first episode of hypercalcaemia, the cause needs to be ascertained.
- The best long-term management of hypercalcaemia is management of the underlying disorder.

Further reading

Oxford Textbook of Medicine, vol 2, p. 375
Oxford Textbook of Palliative Medicine, 3rd ed. pp. 688–690
Oxford Handbook of Palliative Care, pp. 365, 768

Respiratory problems

☼ Community-acquired pneumonia

- Pneumonia is any infection of the lung parenchyma.
- For most people, the source of infection is the oropharynx or aerobic Gram-negative bacilli from the upper GIT.
- Rarely, pneumonia is caused by airborne organisms (tuberculosis, *Legionella*, and Q fever) or from extra-pulmonary sites.
- In life-limiting illnesses, progressive immobility, pre-existing lung disease, diabetes, and increasing age are a significant factors in developing pneumonia.

History

Pneumonia may present with **sudden onset of fevers, purulent sputum**, and, at times, **pleuritic chest** pain. Less typical presentations include an insidious onset of influenza-like symptoms (myalgias and arthralgias, headache, and fatigue) and dry cough. The degree of breathlessness varies widely. For many people symptoms of sepsis dominate over respiratory compromise.

In someone with a life-limiting illness, clinicians need to distinguish between:

- an infection complicating an overall deterioration (often seen as a terminal event)
- a pneumonic process in someone who is otherwise still relatively well.

Physical examination

Acutely, people will have **fever and tachycardia**, and may be hypotensive or obtunded when severely ill. A person may have evidence of **central cyanosis** (lips or ear lobes) with **significant respiratory compromise**.

On examination over the affected side, there may be decreased expansion, percussion note, vocal resonance, and air entry with coarse crackles. In less typical presentations of pneumonia, abnormal physical findings may be surprisingly few except for scattered rales or first onset of wheezing in an adult.

Investigations and management

Prognosis measured in hours to days prior to the onset of this problem (symptom control)

For someone at the end-of-life who intercurrently develops a clinical pneumonia, **no further investigations are warranted**.

Symptom control is as for **dyspnoea** (p. 24) and any associated **confusion** (p. 28). Reverse any symptomatic **hypoxaemia** with supplemental oxygen. **Treat fever** with paracetamol or NSAIDS (p. 46). Ensure adequate hydration in the setting of sepsis.

Prognosis measured in weeks prior to the onset of this problem (in addition to symptom control)

CXR will demonstrate pulmonary infiltrates in most people with pneumonia. People in whom infiltrates may not be seen include those early in the course of the infection and those who are not mounting an immune response, including people with agranulocytosis. Multicentric infiltrates suggests haematogenous spread. Diffuse infiltrates suggest an atypical organism, including *Pneumocystis carinii* or a viral pathogen.

Cavitation can occur with pathogens including oral anaerobes, *Staphylococcus aureus, Streptococcus pneumoniae, Mycobacterium tuberculosis, Nocardia*, and fungal infections including *Histoplasma capsulatum, Coccidiodes immitis*, and *Blastomyces dermatiditis*. Fungal infections can cause hilar lymphadenopathy and pleural effusions.

FBC should be obtained for the WCC with differential. In established pneumonia, the failure to mount a leucocytosis is a poor prognostic factor. Take **blood cultures.**

Treating pneumonia with antibiotics may help reduce delirium, cough, and purulent sputum in some people. For people who are relatively well and mobile without significant sepsis or haemodynamic compromise, consider oral out-patient-based care. Oral amoxycillin–clavulinic acid twice daily will cover most *Streptococcus pneumoniae, Haemophilus influenzae, Moraxella catarrhalis,* and anaerobes. Macrolides such as oral roxithromycin 300 mg daily for 7 days will cover *Mycoplasma pneumoniae, Chlamydia pneumoniae,* and *Legionella pneumophilia.*

Prognosis measured in months to years prior to the onset of this problem (in addition to 'Prognosis measured in week')

Serum needs to be sent if there is a question of atypical organisms including *Mycoplasma* or *Legionella* infections.

Sputum culture will yield a pathogenic organism in less than 50 per cent of cases.

If there are risk factors for HIV infection, HIV status should be established after appropriate counselling and consent. *Pneumocystis carinii* should be specifically sought on an induced sputum.

In someone who is otherwise functionally well, there may be a case for fibre-optic bronchoscopy to obtain lower respiratory tract secretions in someone not responding to treatment.

For people who need to be hospitalized because of systemic or respiratory compromise, a second- or third-generation cephalosporin will cover a broad range of organisms including *Staphylococcus aureus*. If there is concern about anaerobic Gram-negative bacilli, metronidazole should be added. Atypical organisms will be covered by macrolides.

Poor outcomes are associated with cancer, organ failure, increasing age or debility, and infections with influenza virus, pneumococcal pneumonitis, or *Legionella*.

Other pneumonias

- In-patient acquired pneumonia
- Pneumonia in the immunocompromised
- Pneumonia after aspiration.

In-patient acquired pneumonia

- There are a series of organisms that are more frequently encountered in people who develop pneumonia in hospital or in residential care settings. Organisms in these settings tend to be more pathogenic, and people tend to be sicker.

- Organisms more likely to be encountered include enteric Gram-negative bacilli, Pseudomonas aeruginosa, Staphylococcus aureus, and oral anaerobes.

Pneumonia in the immunocompromised

- In the elderly, Haemophilus influenzae, Legionella pneumophilia, and Moraxella catarrhalis are the most common organisms. In the institutionalized elderly, Pseudomonas aeruginosa and Staphylococcus aureus are more frequently encountered than in the community at large.
- In people with hypogammaglobulinaemia (or a person who had not been immunized after splenectomy), encapsulated organisms such as Streptococcus pneumoniae and Haemophilus influenzae need to be considered. The malnutrition of cachexia and protein-losing enteropathies also compromise humoral immunity.
- Where HIV levels in the community are high, Mycobacterium tuberculosis is often encountered. Pneumocystis carinii and cytomegalovirus (where the clinical picture may be predominantly of extra-pulmonary symptoms with a dry cough and increasing shortness of breath) are also encountered.

Pneumonia associated with aspiration

There are potentially three sources of aspiration: oral flora, food, or acidic gastric contents.

Aspiration pneumonia develops in an insidious way. More than 50 per cent of adults will normally have measurable micro-aspiration of upper aerodigestive tract contents while sleeping. This is worsened with gingival disease.

Oral flora that can cause lung infections include Gram-positive Actinomyces species, Gram-negative Prevotella melaninogenica, Fusobacterium, Bacteroides species other than Bacteroides fragilis, and anaerobic cocci including Gram-positive Peptostreptococcus and Gram-negative Veillonella.

For aspiration of oral contents, X-ray changes are most frequently in the basilar segments of the lower lobes if upright when aspirating or, if supine, in the postero-basilar segments of the upper lobe or the superior segment of the lower lobe.

Food is usually aspirated when consciousness is impaired or with a neurological cause for dysphagia. A post-obstruction bacterial pneumonia can develop in people with tumour obstructing large airways. In people with dysphagia, the introduction of NG feeding does not decrease the risk of aspiration pneumonia.

Aspiration of gastric contents can cause a chemical pneumonitis, with diffuse changes on X-ray occurring rapidly after the aspiration.

Further reading

Oxford Textbook of Medicine, Vol. 2, pp. 1357–1376
Oxford Textbook of Palliative Medicine, p. 863
Oxford Handbook of Palliative Care, p. 296

✛ **Pleural effusion**

- Most people with a pleural effusion experience this as an asymptomatic finding on CXR.
- The nature of the pleural fluid helps to define the underlying pathology and therapeutic interventions available.

Causes of pleural effusion

	Frequently encountered causes	**Less frequently encountered causes**
Cancer (exudate)	Any primary or secondary carcinoma (lung, breast cancer, lymphoma)	Mesothelioma
End-stage organ failure (transudate)	Cardiac or hepatic failure	Nephrotic syndrome
Intercurrent illnesses (exudate)	Pneumonia Pulmonary embolus	Connective tissue diseases

History

Increasing shortness of breath on exertion is the most common presentation. Often people will note that they are unable to lie on the side opposite to the effusion. For most people the progression of symptoms with a pleural effusion is subtle.

Sudden onset of shortness of breath in the presence of a pleural effusion should flag exclusion of other pathology: pneumonia, pulmonary embolus, or obstruction of a large airway.

Physical examination

On observation, check for **central cyanosis** (tongue or ear lobes). Is the trachea deviated away from the side of the effusion?

Record respiratory and pulse rate. When checking blood pressure check for evidence of pulsus paradoxus (drop of >10 mmHg in systolic blood pressure on inspiration). Given the risk of concomitant pericardial fluid, check for jugular venous engorgement. **Decreased expansion of the affected side may be seen together with dullness to percussion, decreased vocal resonance, and decreased or absent air entry**.

Investigations and management

Prognosis measured in hours to days prior to onset of this problem (symptom control)

Pleural effusions are commonly encountered at the end-of-life. **The only reason to consider bedside drainage is that the person had rapidly re-accumulating fluid and symptomatic benefit from previous drainage**. At the bedside, check **pulse oximetry**. **Oxygen** may be of benefit in people with significant hypoxaemia.

Energy conservation should be used to minimize breathlessness.

People who are opioid naive and are breathless should be offered low-dose opioids. People already on opioids should be offered a 30–50 per cent increase on baseline. Anxiety may benefit from relaxation techniques or anxiolytics.

Prognosis measured in weeks prior to the onset of this problem (in addition to symptom control)

In the community or in hospital, a **CXR** can define the effusion and any underlying lung pathology such as pneumonia or a wedge-shaped pulmonary infarct from an embolus. A **chest ultrasound** can define the size of the effusion and whether there is loculation, and provide direct guidance for drainage.

If symptomatic, consider drainage to a level that breathlessness is relieved. People occasionally experience re-expansion pulmonary oedema in the hours after evacuation of pleural fluid with sudden respiratory decompensation.

Prognosis measured in months to years prior to the onset of this problem (in addition to prognosis measured in weeks)

Thoracic CT can better define underlying lung pathology.

Perform a diagnostic tap and send pleural fluid for laboratory evaluation. **Pleural fluid** should have a **cell count** (>5000/µl suggests pulmonary embolism or neoplasm), **cytology, protein levels** (ratio of pleural to serum levels >0.5 consistent with exudate), **lactate dehydrogenase** (ratio of pleural: to serum levels >0.6 consistent with a transudate), **microscopy** (including a search for acid fast bacilli), and **culture** (including tuberculosis if the cause of the effusion is unknown).

If the effusion is malignant, consider drainage through a formal chest tube, followed by pleurodesis if the cavity can be made dry. Alternatively a video-assisted thoracoscopy may be indicated. If the effusion is loculated (de novo or as a result of previous attempts at pleurodesis), use ultrasound guidance.

If the lung fails to re-expand, further drainage is not indicated unless normal lung tissue is being compressed.

Further reading

Oxford Textbook of Medicine, Vol. 2, pp. 1513–1515.
Oxford Textbook of Palliative Medicine, p. 262.
Oxford Handbook of Palliative Care, pp. 302–303.

☼ Empyema

- Pus in the pleural space may occur as a complication of a para-pneumonic process, or as a complication of previous instrumentation of the pleural space.
- Pus loculates rapidly, and if there is a suggestion of sepsis within the pleural space, drain the fluid as soon as possible.

Causes of empyema

	Frequently encountered causes	Less frequently encountered causes
Cancer	Malignant pleural effusions	
Intercurrent illnesses	Para-pneumonic process	TB (depending on where in the world)
	Uraemia	Bronchiectasis

History
Although people with an effusion may complain of breathlessness, there needs to be an index of suspicion in a person with a pneumonic process and pleural effusion or a person with a pleural effusion, fever, and previous invasive procedures involving the pleural space.

Physical examination
Physical findings will reflect the fluid within the pleural cavity.

Evidence of sepsis with systemic compromise should be sought. Fever, hypotension, tachycardia, and hypoxaemia should be regularly sought. An underlying pneumonia may be difficult to diagnose, but needs to be considered when there is obstruction of a large airway.

Investigations and management
Prognosis measured in hours to days prior to onset of this problem (symptom control)
Treat fever with paracetamol or NSAIDs. Definitive treatment is not possible in people who are frail and near death.

The onset and symptoms may not be as pronounced for people with anaerobic infections. Severe influenza-like symptoms may predominate in people at the end-of-life with an empyema who are not well enough for either local or systemic treatment.

Prognosis measured in weeks prior to the onset of this problem (in addition to symptom control)
Pleural fluid should be sent for urgent **microscopy** including **Gram stain** if an empyema is suspected. Diagnosis without positive Gram stain is problematic.

Culture of pleural fluid, including TB, should be done. Aerobic and anaerobic organisms each account for 50 per cent of empyemas. Aerobic organisms frequently include *Streptococcus pneumoniae*, *Staphylococcus* *aureus*, Gram-negative bacilli include *Enterobacter*, *Klebsiella* and *Proteus* species. Anaerobic organisms include *Actinomyces* species, *Prevotella melaninogenica*, *Fusobacterium*, *Peptostreptococcus* and *Veillonella*.

Pleural fluid may have a glucose level of <50 mg/dl and a pH >0.15 below arterial pH (or an absolute level <7.0) in the presence of an empyema. Urgently drain the pleural space with a large-bore chest drain after excluding a coagulopathy.

Prognosis measured in months to years prior to the onset of this problem (in addition to 'Prognosis measured in weeks')

Ensure adequate close monitoring while arranging for the drainage of the chest cavity with a chest tube. Ensure that a large-bore cannula is in place. Commence empiric antibiotics with a third-generation cephalosporin such as ceftriaxone 1 g IV daily and an aminoglycoside such as gentamicin 3–5 mg/kg/day IV while awaiting definitive cultures.

If already loculated, consider use of streptokinase to break down fibrin bands. If there is an established loculation, consult with the cardiothoracic service to consider video-assisted thoracoscopy.

Further reading

Oxford Textbook of Medicine, Vol. 2, pp. 1517–1518.
Oxford Handbook of Palliative Care, p. 582.

☼ **Pneumothorax**

- In people with a life-limiting illness, a pneumothorax is rarely a primary event. Secondary pneumothoraces may be spontaneous or traumatic.
- A pneumothorax is a more significant problem in the palliative setting because of pre-existing lung compromise.

Causes of pneumothorax

	Frequently encountered causes	**Less frequently encountered causes**
Cancer	Any lung cancer, following lung biopsy or pleural aspiration	Pathological rib fracture Oesophageal rupture
End-stage organ failure	Chronic obstructive pulmonary disease (rupture of bullae)	Cystic fibrosis
Inter-current illnesses	Placement of a central venous catheter	Mechanical ventilation *Pneumocystis carinii* pneumonia

History

- Most people with a life-limiting illness have a pneumothorax found as an incidental finding on CXR. It is often not associated with chest pain or any other discomfort.
- People may initially experience some mild shortness of breath on exertion or pleuritic pain on deep inspiration.
- **If the person has respiratory symptoms, urgently exclude a tension pneumothorax.**

Physical examination

Tracheal shift away from the midline on the affected side suggests a tension pneumothorax with signs of respiratory and subsequent cardiac compromise (tachypnoea, tachycardia, hypotension, desaturation). **Absent air entry** on the affected side supports this diagnosis. **Urgently decompress the chest with a chest drain on the affected side**.

Physical signs include reduced expansion on the affected side together with decreased air entry. Hyper-resonance is difficult to elicit. Vocal resonance may be increased.

In a pneumothorax secondary to instrumentation, physical signs may be absent or subtle. A high index of suspicion is needed, especially in people who have had invasive thoracic procedures.

Investigations and management

Prognosis measured in hours to days prior to onset of this problem (symptom control)

Assess for respiratory compromise. **Supplemental oxygen** should be administered while the extent of the problem is being defined. **Anxiety and dyspnoea can be prominent. Any significant pneumothorax is likely to be a terminal event in people at the end-of-life.**

*Prognosis measured in weeks prior to the onset of this problem
(in addition to symptom control)*

A **CXR** will demonstrate the degree of lung collapse. It is also the crucial way to follow progress. A pneumothorax that is increasing in size needs to be followed closely. **Thoracic CT** will help to define any underlying pathology when the person has been stabilized.

When intrapleural pressure is above atmospheric pressure and there is free gas in the pleural space, the person has a **tension pneumothorax**. Impaired cardiac output and hypoxaemia rapidly cause death. The decision to treat will need to be made with the person who has a life-limiting illness.

A large-bore intercostal needle should be introduced into the pleural space urgently and replaced with an intercostal drain as soon as possible.

The other indication for a chest drain is if a pneumothorax is larger than 30 per cent or expanding.

In people with a small post-biopsy pneumothorax, observation is usually sufficient. Air will be reabsorbed slowly from the pleural surface if the original leak is sealed. Simple aspiration is reserved for people with a primary spontaneous pneumothorax.

*Prognosis measured in months to years prior to the onset of this
problem (in addition to prognosis measured in weeks)*

In someone where a chest tube is draining a pneumothorax and the lung (not tethered by scar tissue) has not re-expanded within a week, consider thoracoscopy.

Further reading

Oxford Textbook of Medicine, Vol. 2, pp. 1519–1520.
Oxford Textbook of Palliative Medicine, p. 910.
Oxford Handbook of Palliative Care, p. 582.

⚠ **Tracheo-oesophageal fistula**

- The most frequently encountered acquired form of tracheo-oesophageal fistula is from oesophageal cancer, although in a small number of people it may be due to violent vomiting.

History

- **Dysphagia** is the most common presentation of oesophageal carcinoma. A tracheo-oesophageal fistula is an uncommon presentation of a primary oesophageal malignancy but more frequently a later complication.
- **Coughing after liquid** intake must be distinguished from upper aero-digestive tract dysphagia.
- The predominant presentation is with **severe retrosternal** pain, worsened by swallowing or deep breathing. The pain may be interscapular as the oesophagus lies within the posterior third of the mediastinum.
- **Fever** or other systemic signs of sepsis suggest mediastinal infection (including potentially abscess formation) or a pneumonic process (chemical or infective).
- With reflux or vomiting, acidic gastric contents may be expressed into the mediastinum.

Physical examination

The physical examination may be apparently normal in the presence of a small fistula.

When the oesophagus has ruptured, there may be findings of a pneumothorax (p. 272) and subcutaneous emphysema at the base of the neck. Findings may reflect aspiration and ensuing inflammation of the airspaces of the lower lobes by a pneumonic process (p. 266) There may be sternal tenderness in the presence of mediastinitis. Check for systemic evidence of sepsis: blood pressure, pulse, temperature. Check pulse oximetry.

Investigations and management

Prognosis measured in hours to days prior to onset of this problem (symptom control)

Stop oral intake and ensure adequate parenteral fluids. Consider a NG tube to empty gastric contents as a transient measure.

Adequate pain relief is required. For many people pain is the predominant and overwhelming symptom. Use maximal acid suppression with a PPI. Opioids are frequently required for the pain of mediastinitis.

Prognosis measured in weeks prior to the onset of this problem (in addition to symptom control)

Although a **CXR** may show abnormalities, a **thoracic CT scan** of the chest is the best way to demonstrate free mediastinal or pleural air. A **gastrograffin swallow** will delineate the level of perforation. With a high index of suspicion, **oesophagoscopy** is the investigation of choice as there may be the possibility of placing a stent to block the fistula in the same procedure. Most people with a life-limiting illness will not tolerate a definitive surgical procedure.

Check for evidence of sepsis. Look at the differential WCC and perform blood cultures if sepsis is suspected. If there is pneumonia or mediastinal sepsis, broad-spectrum antibiotics need to include cover for oral anaerobes (p. 266).

Prognosis measured in months to years prior to the onset of this problem in addition to 'prognosis measured in weeks'

As tracheo-oesophageal fistulae are most frequently encountered in oesophageal cancer, explore all definitive options for treatment.

Further reading

Oxford Textbook of Medicine, Vol. 2, pp. 630, 638.

☠ Mediastinitis

- Inflammation or infection within the mediastinal space is an event secondary to a small number of insults.
- The onset of this may be sudden and present in a person who is *in extremis*.

Causes of mediastinitis (rare clinical presentation)

	Frequently encountered causes	**Less frequently encountered causes**
Cancer	Perforation of an oesophageal cancer	Perforation during an upper digestive tract endoscopic procedure, insertion of a Blakemore tube, or during endoscopic oesophageal dilatation

History

People with mediastinitis are extremely ill. Symptoms include pain and shortness of breath. The pain will depend on which third of the mediastinum is affected. As the oesophagus runs through the posterior third, pain is often referred to the person's back, neck, arms, or shoulders. People may describe the pain as being 'constricting', akin to an acute coronary syndrome.

Post-surgically, people may present with acute sepsis or a purulent discharge from a sternotomy or thoracoscopy scar.

Pneumo-mediastinum can occur with the rupture of the oesophagus or airways at any level, or air tracking from the neck or peritoneal cavity.

Physical examination

Check whether the person is **systemically unwell**: pulse, blood pressure, temperature, and oxygen saturation. In the post-procedure setting, there may be signs of local infection with tenderness, erythema, warmth, and a discharge. If mediastinitis affects the middle third, there may be click with each heartbeat.

In the presence of a pneumo-mediastinum, there may be subcutaneous emphysema that generally tracks to the neck.

Investigations and management

Prognosis measured in hours to days prior to onset of this problem (symptom control)

Pain is still the major problem with mediastinitis. Use of opioid analgesia is necessary to provide adequate analgesia. Fever may predominate.

Prognosis measured in weeks prior to the onset of this problem (in addition to symptom control)

On **CXR** there may be evidence of the widening of the mediatinum and evidence of free gas. The definitive examination for mediastinal pathology is **CT**. With the working diagnosis of a ruptured oesophagus, a **contrast swallowing study** may be helpful.

Check **FBC** for neutrophilia and take **blood cultures**.

For post-surgical mediastinitis, drain any collection and debride tissue with marginal viability. Use aggressive doses of parenteral antibiotics with broad-spectrum coverage including anaerobic cover (p. 48). Monitor carefully until the person is stable.

Prognosis measured in months to years prior to the onset of this problem (in addition to prognosis measured in weeks)

In the palliative or supportive care setting, a **video-assisted mediastino-scopy** is rarely required. Surgical repair of an oesophageal perforation is rarely an option for people with a life-limiting illness. An attempt at stenting and treating mediastinitis with antibiotics will be the definitive procedure for most people. Post-surgical mediastinitis is a serious com-plication, with a mortality rate still approaching 20 per cent.

Further reading

Oxford Textbook of Medicine, Vol. 2, p. 638.

☼ Large-airway problems

- Obstruction from growth within the bronchial tree or external compression can narrow the lumen of large airways.

Causes of compromise to large airways

	Frequently encountered causes	**Less frequently encountered causes**
Cancer	Primary or secondary lung cancers, especially broncho-alveolar carcinoma (with potential for trans-bronchial spread)	Extrinsic compression by malignant mediastinal lymph nodes
Intercurrent illnesses		Bronchial adenomas, sarcoidosis (only 80 per cent have bilateral hilar lymphadenopathy)

History

Symptoms of large-airway obstruction include **cough**, which in the case of adenomas may be present for many years. **Haemoptysis** can frequently occur. **Wheeze, stridor, and progressive dyspnoea** may be the predominant finding. (Inspiratory stridor tends to suggest supraglottic pathology and expiratory stridor subglottic problems.)

Recurrent or refractory pneumonia (distal to partial or total obstruction) is frequently encountered.

Tracheal obstruction is most commonly from enlarged mediastinal nodes that may cause varying degrees of oesophageal obstruction, recurrent laryngeal nerve paralysis (hoarse voice), or phrenic nerve involvement (sudden worsening in dyspnoea as a hemi-diaphragm fails to contribute to respiratory effort).

With a life-limiting illness, it is rare that large-airway obstruction will be new pathology. Rather, it is more likely to be progression of documented disease.

Physical examination

Physical findings should reflect the level at which the airway is compromised. Horner's syndrome (small pupil, partial ptosis, ipsilateral loss of sweating, and enophthalmus (loss of the tarsal muscles)) will occur with damaged cervical sympathetic chain.

Do the lungs expand symmetrically (a relatively small airway may be affected) or is expansion largely absent on one side (a main bronchus is obstructed)? Percussion and careful auscultation may help localization. With loss of a hemi-diaphragm in phrenic nerve lesions, the spleen or liver may appear unusually high.

Investigations and management

Prognosis measured in hours to days prior to the onset of this problem (symptom control)

Ensure **adequate oxygenation** and use supplemental oxygen if there is hypoxaemia. Most symptoms are related to **cough or dyspnoea**. Cough can be particularly problematic. A combination of opioids and anxiolytics will help with these symptoms.

Prognosis measured in weeks prior to the onset of this problem (in addition to symptom control)

CXR will demonstrate any collapse or consolidation. It may also demonstrate any lymphadenopathy. A **chest CT** will further define pathology.

Bronchoscopy will define the pathology. Bronchoscopic stenting may help with extrinsic compression of airways and be of use if there is no post-obstruction collapse/consolidation. (If consolidation is already evident, stenting will not produce re-expansion of the lung.) Laser ablation of endobronchial tumours or their removal can be offered at endoscopy.

Bronchomalacia can occur after lung transplantation. Because the blood supply to the bronchi is not directly restored at surgery, the anastomosis relies on retrograde blood flow. Anastamotic leaks or later stenosis are frequently encountered. Bronchoscopic stenting may help with some anastamotic problems. A bronchial fistula can occur if the anastamosis breaks down.

Further reading

Oxford Textbook of Medicine, Vol. 2, pp. 1404–1408.
Oxford Textbook of Palliative Medicine, pp. 262, 598–599
Oxford Handbook of Palliative Care, p. 359

☠ Haemoptysis

- Haemoptysis is a feared complication of many end-of-life respiratory illnesses.

Causes of haemoptysis

	Frequently encountered causes	**Less frequently encountered causes**
Cancer	Primary lung cancer Cancers of the upper aero-digestive tract	
Intercurrent illnesses	Bronchiectasis	TB
	Pulmonary infarction	Fungus ball
	Rupture of mucosal blood vessel with vigorous coughing	Lung abscess
		Mitral stenosis
		Acute left ventricular failure
		Primary pulmonary hypertension

History
Bleeding can occur at any time in people with lung cancer. There will often be no sentinel bleed. Volume of bleeding is difficult to estimate, but in extensive bleeding, the blood appears bright red and at times frothy. Bleeding causing any difficulty in breathing is significant.

Define the likely mechanism of the bleed. For example, haemoptysis that arises from pulmonary embolism is an important diagnosis even with a life-limiting illness.

Other, bleeding that may mimic haemoptysis includes upper GIT bleeding, when both coughing and vomiting are present, and bleeding from the nasopharynx. Secondary malignancies in the lungs rarely generate haemoptysis.

Physical examination
Establish the **person's haemodynamic status**: blood pressure, pulse, and oxygen saturation. Look for other evidence of bleeding or bruising. Look for the cause of haemoptysis: bronchitis, pneumonia, pulmonary infarction from pulmonary embolus, underlying mitral stenosis, or evidence of left ventricular failure.

Investigations and management
Prognosis measured in hours to days prior to the onset of this problem (symptom control)
With significant haemoptysis, **stop any medications that may be adding to bleeding**: anticoagulants, NSAIDs, and clopidogrel. **Consider vitamin K for people who have been on warfarin**, or, if there are no contraindications, **oral tranexamic acid** 500mg QID.

Haemoptysis is frightening. Everyone around the bed is likely to be frightened. In someone for whom this is the terminal event and where active measures are not to be pursued, provide adequate analgesia and sedation with a combination of opioids and benzodiazepines (intravenous if necessary) as death from bleeding is mostly from obliteration of airways with irritative blood. Red or green linen will reduce the visual impact of bleeding.

Prognosis measured in weeks prior to the onset of this problem (in addition to symptom control)

If seeking a distinction between bleeding from lung and stomach, check **pH** as respiratory bleeding will be slightly alkaline.

Check **coagulation studies**, looking for coagulopathies including DIC (low platelets, prolonged activated partial thromboplastin time, red cell fragments which may be present on a blood film, and raised fibrinogen degradation products) (p. 168).

A **CXR** may show evidence of lobar pneumonia, lobar collapse (because of a more proximal intraluminal lesion obstructing that lobe), or the wedge-shaped peripheral lesion of a pulmonary infarct.

In people with more than streaks of blood in sputum, a **bronchoscopy** should be carried out on a semi-urgent basis if there is no explanation for the bleeding. This may also be therapeutic as there is the ability to use a laser to diathermy a bleeding vessel.

Prognosis measured in months to years prior to the onset of this problem (in addition to prognosis measured in weeks)

Most bleeding from the lungs stops spontaneously. Larger volume bleeds (>500 ml in 24 hs) are less likely to stop without intervention. If the bleeding is from primary lung cancer, explore local treatment options: laser coagulation, external beam radiotherapy, or brachytherapy.

Rarely, selective intubation to isolate a lobe where there is bleeding may preserve the rest of the lung' function. Bronchial artery catheterization and selective embolization is an option for ongoing low-level bleeding. Open surgery is rarely an option.

Further reading

Oxford Textbook of Medicine, Vol. 2, p. 1284.
Oxford Textbook of Palliative Medicine, pp. 610–611, 251.
Oxford Handbook of Palliative Care, pp. 404–405.

① Pneumonitis

- Pneumonitis occurs most commonly as an iatrogenic complication of radiotherapy or chemotherapy, infection, or connective tissue diseases.

Causes of pneumonitis

	Frequently encountered causes	**Less frequently encountered causes**
Cancer	Chemotherapy (acutely)	
	Radiotherapy (2–3 months after treatment)	
Intercurrent illenesses	Rheumatoid arthritis	Systemic lupus erythematosus (SLE)
	Occupational lung disease including asbestosis	

History

People with pneumonitis present with **cough and dyspnoea**, and are often systemically unwell with **fever and malaise**.

The syndrome may mimic an atypical pneumonia in time course, presentation, and physical findings. An acute clinical course may follow exposure to a number of chemotherapeutic agents including cyclophosphamide, methotrexate, gemcitabine, bleomycin, busulphan, chlorambucil, taxanes, and temazolamide.

Lung signs and symptoms are delayed until some months after treatment with radiotherapy. Unlike other complications of radiotherapy, the respiratory findings can be more widespread than the irradiated area. Mucous plugs with fibrous tissue (bronchiolitis obliterans with organizing pneumonia (BOOP)) may be seen.

Rheumatoid arthritis can have both fibrosing alveolitis and interstitial fibrosis. Along with SLE and drug-induced pneumonitis, these changes predominate in the lower lobes.

Physical examination

The physical examination may be **normal throughout the clinical course**. Look for central cyanosis on lips or ear lobes. Clubbing suggests that there is long-standing pathology. Look for evidence of respiratory distress including tachypnoea at rest or on minimal exertion. Fine late inspiratory crackles may be heard in the affected area.

Right-sided heart strain may manifest as overt failure or evidence of increased pressures on the right side of the heart with a loud pulmonary component of the second heart sound.

Investigations and management
Prognosis measured in hours to days prior to onset of this problem (symptom control)

The breathlessness caused is often progressive and associated with significant fear as function worsens and breathlessness intensifies. Adequate psychological support and relaxation techniques are an important adjunct to the pharmacological interventions that are offered. Energy conservation techniques are an integral part of management.

Check oxygenation. Exclude an atypical pneumonia that may mimic the presentation. Discontinue the offending agent if the pneumonitis is medication related.

Prognosis measured in weeks prior to the onset of this problem (in addition to symptom control)

The **CXR** may show little change early in the course of the clinical presentation. The pattern of interstitial changes will confirm clinical suspicions. Mild hypoxaemia with normal or low partial pressure of carbon dioxide is seen on **arterial blood gases**. **Chest CT** may delineate the extent of lung changes. In long-standing changes, a restrictive pattern may be seen on **pulmonary function tests** and secondary polycythaemia may be present on **FBC**.

Glucocorticoids may play a role in reducing local inflammation and reducing the intensity of symptoms.

Prognosis measured in months to years prior to the onset of this problem (in addition to prognosis measured in weeks)

If beneficial, glucocorticoids should subsequently be weaned very slowly. Treat any underlying connective tissue disorder.

Further reading

Oxford Textbook of Medicine Vol. 2, pp. 1506–1507
Oxford Textbook of Palliative Medicine, p. 241
Oxford Handbook of Palliative Care, p. 127

① **Lymphangitis carcinomatosis**

- The blockage of lung lymphatics by tumour creates the clinical presentation of lymphangitis carcinomatosis.

Malignancies associated with lymphangitis carcinomatosis

	Frequently encountered causes	**Less frequently encountered causes**
Cancer	Adenocarcinoma of the lung or breast	Other malignancies

History

People with lymphangitis present with shortness of breath which can mimic pulmonary oedema, an atypical pneumonia, or a pulmonary embolus. Progressively severe breathlessness is the most frequently encountered clinical course. Hypoxaemia can be profound and develop rapidly.

There may be little else to find on history, physical examination, or imaging.

Physical examination

Early in the clinical course, the physical examination may be normal. Look for central cyanosis of the lips or ear lobes. Look for evidence of respiratory distress including tachypnoea at rest or on minimal exertion.

Investigations and management

Prognosis measured in hours to days prior to the onset of this problem (symptom control)

Exclude an atypical pneumonia that may mimic the presentation.

The major symptomatic intervention is **relief of breathlessness**. Oxygen may be of benefit early in the course of lymphangitis carcinomatosis. **Opioids and anxiolytics** will provide symptomatic relief.

Prognosis measured in weeks prior to the onset of this problem (in addition to symptom control)

CXR may show hilar enlargement with fan-shaped opacities radiating, reflecting tumour spread through lymphatic channels. Kerley B lines may be visible. **Sputum cytology** may be positive for malignant cells. Check pulse oximetry.

Unless the underlying malignancy is responsive to chemotherapy, little is likely to reverse this problem. There are case reports of glucocorticoids offering some early symptomatic benefit.

Prognosis measured in months to years prior to the onset of this problem (in addition to prognosis measured in weeks)

Transthoracic or occasionally transbronchial biopsy may be used to confirm the diagnosis of lymphangitis carcinomatosis.

People with a primary breast cancer with submaximal systemic treatment should be offered hormone therapy for oestrogen- or progesterone-positive tumours or systemic cytotoxic chemotherapy to which the cancer has not been previously exposed. The presence of lymphangitis carcinomatosis is a very poor prognostic sign, with median survival measured in weeks.

Further reading

Oxford Textbook of Medicine, Vol. 2, p. 1543.
Oxford Textbook of Palliative Medicine, p. 599

Genitourological disorders

! **Upper urinary tract infections**

- Upper urinary tract infections include acute pyelonephritis and prostatitis.
- Upper urinary tract infections are generally parenchymal, whilst lower tract problems tend to be limited to the mucosa.
- Urinary tract infections may be divided into complicated (instrumentation, indwelling catheters, or structural abnormalities) and uncomplicated.

Causes of upper urinary tract infections
Pyelonephritis
Ascending infection
Structural abnormalities of the urinary tract
Immunodeficiency
Complicated lower urinary tract infections
Chronic illness
Haematogenous spread of infection to the kidneys
Prostatitis
Spontaneous
Urinary catheters

History

- People with **acute pyelonephritis present with an acute onset of fever, rigor, flank pain, and dysuria.**
- **Prostatitis presents with fever, rigor, and dysuria, but is associated with lower back or perineal pain.** These people may develop acute urinary retention.

Physical examination

These people may be very unwell. They may be **febrile or hypothermic, with a thready tachycardia and hypotension.**

Patients with **pyelonephritis often have tenderness to palpation over the renal angle on the affected side**. Abdominal examination may reveal generalized tenderness with guarding.

People with **prostatitis will display an extremely tender and soft prostate.** Caution must be exercised in examining these men as massage of an inflamed prostate may lead to bacteraemia.

Investigations and management

Prognosis measured in hours to days prior to the onset of this problem (symptom control)

Despite the very limited prognosis of this group, it may be possible to improve comfort by ensuring adequate hydration (SC or IVI fluids) and

administration of appropriate antibiotics. This may be by a single dose of gentamicin 2 mg/kg and ceftriaxone 1 g which may help to control fever and rigor. Other simple interventions to control fever include regular sustained release paracetamol (500 mg rectally four times daily, 1 g orally four times daily, or 1330 mg Q8h) or NSAIDs (Ketorolac 10 mg SC every 8 hs, indomethacin 100 mg rectally twice daily).

Prognosis measured in weeks prior to the onset of this problem (in addition to symptom control)

The diagnosis of pyelonephritis is based on a combination of history and **the presence of an elevated WCC, raised inflammatory markers** (ESR, CRP), and **positive urine cultures**.

   The diagnosis of prostatitis is made on a combination of clinical features (fever, dysuria, and a tender prostate) and **positive urine cultures**.

   People with pyelonephritis may be managed with oral antibiotics (amoxicillin–clavulianic acid every 12 hs for 10 days) if they do not have septicaemia or complicated infection (instrumentation, indwelling urinary catheter). With nausea and vomiting, hypotension, or a complicated infection, management includes fluid resuscitation and parenteral antibiotics. Cover *Escherichia.coli* with ceftriaxone 1 g IV, daily and adjust antibiotics when urine and blood cultures are available.

   Acute prostatitis is likely to be due to *E. coli* or Klebsiella. Cover with trimethoprim 300 mg daily for 14 days or cefalexin 500 mg every 12 hs for 14 days.

Prognosis measured in months to years prior to the onset of this problem (in addition to the above)

Uncomplicated pyelonephritis should resolve. With anatomical abnormalities, long-term use of antibiotics may be necessary in the pallative setting.

   Prostatitis carries a reasonably high rate of relapse with the development of resistant organisms. This dictates the need for long-term antibiotics and prostatectomy.

   Both these disorders may be associated with pain nausea and vomiting. Attention must be paid to hydration, analgesia, and antiemetic therapy. Significant morbidity may occur in the presence of structural abnormalities.

Further reading

Oxford Textbook of Medicine, Vol. 3, pp. 420–424.
Oxford Handbook of Palliative Care, p. 322–326.

① **Lower urinary tract infections**

- Lower urinary tract infections refer to infections of the bladder and urethra.

Causes of lower urinary tract infections
Urethritis
Ascending infection
Instrumentation of the urinary tract
Indwelling catheters
Additional causes of cystitis
Prostatitis
Fistula formation

History

Cystitis tends to be more symptomatic in people describing fever, marked dysuria, haematuria, frequency, and the passage of small amounts of urine only. There may be associated suprapubic or lower back pain. In considering a fistula, a history of pneumaturia or passage of faecal matter through the urethra should be sought (p. 300).

Abrupt onset of symptoms is most likely to be due to *Escherichia coli* in the community, and either an *E. coli* or staphylococcal infection when acquired in hospital. A more gradual onset of symptoms suggests *Chlamydia* or gonococcal infection in people who are sexually active. Men may develop urethral discharge.

People with urethritis usually present with milder symptoms. Dysuria is reported, and some people may have low-grade fever and urgency of micturition.

Asymptomatic colonization of the urinary tract in someone with an indwelling catheter does not need treatment with antibiotics unless they become systemically unwell.

Physical examination

People may have low-grade fevers and suprapubic tenderness on examination but often nothing else is found.

Investigations and management

Prognosis measured in hours to days prior to the onset of this problem (symptom control)

- Other than a **urinary dipstick, no investigations are indicated**.
- A single dose of **gentamicin (2 mg/kg) IV** and **ceftriaxone 1 g IV** may improve symptoms of pain and fevers.
- Ensure **adequate hydration**.
- A person may be more comfortable with an **indwelling catheter** to avoid sense of urgency and frequency of micturition.
- Ensure **adequate analgesia** (suprapubic pain) and **regular paracetamol** to address fever.

Prognosis measured in weeks or longer prior to the onset of this problem (in addition to symptom control)

- The diagnosis of these disorders is mostly made on urine examination alone. With urethritis, no abnormalities may be detected on urine collection, but cystitis is almost always associated with microscopic haematuria and a positive urine culture.
- These disorders can usually be managed with oral antibiotics alone.
- Check **WCC** with a differential count of neutrophils and **renal function**.
- **Ensure adequate hydration**.
- **Ensure that analgesia** for suprapubic pain and paracetamol for fever is available.

Further reading

Oxford Textbook of Medicine, Vol. 3, pp. 420–424.
Oxford Handbook of Palliative Care, p. 324–326.

⚙ **Urinary tract obstruction**

- Urinary tract obstruction is classified as incomplete or complete, unilateral or bilateral.
- As a result of a complete urinary tract obstruction, a person may develop renal failure (p.184).

Causes of urinary tract obstruction	
Within the lumen of the ureters/urethra	Calculi
	Blood clot
	Papillae sloughing
	Tumour
Within the wall of ureters/urethra	Strictures
	Neurogenic bladder
	Congenital
External pressure on the urinary tract	Tumours
	Retroperitoneal fibrosis
	Granulomatous disease
	Crohn's disease
Other	Surgical trauma

History

- Acute **upper** tract obstruction (kidney and ureters) will present with flank pain that may radiate to the inguinal region or perineum. The pain may increase with fluid intake as a result of pressure from retained urine. There may be deceased or absent urine output.
- An acute **lower** urinary tract obstruction (bladder, urethra) will present with suprapubic pain.
- An incomplete urethral obstruction may be associated with pain, poor stream, or incontinence, and a high risk of infection. Pain may not be present in urinary retention due to a cord lesion (p.204).
- People who are already uraemic may experience drowsiness, nausea, twitching, and itch (p.184).

Physical examination

- **Upper** obstruction may present as loin tenderness or a palpable loin mass only with a significant hydronephrosis.
- **Lower** obstruction may lead to a palpable bladder.
- Check for **fever, hypotension, tachycardia, and dehydration**.
- A **neurological examination** must exclude spinal cord compression (p.204).
- If renal function is deteriorating, this person may already be uraemic, with drowsiness, confusion, and myoclonus.

Investigations and management
Prognosis measured in hours to days prior to the onset of this problem (symptom control)
Further investigations are not indicated at this stage.

People who are not passing urine should have an **indwelling urethral catheter inserted**. Passing an IDC may relieve lower obstructions. In some-one with significant retention, release urine at no more than 500 ml/h to avoid bladder mucosal bleeding. If obstruction is relieved, there may be a large diuresis in which case hydration needs to be carefully monitored. More invasive procedures are not indicated.

People who are anuric will become uraemic and **the symptoms of uraemia must be addressed**. These include nausea (haloperidol 0.5–3.0 mg SC daily), itch (ondansetron wafers 4 mg SL twice daily), and myoclonic jerks (clonazepam 0.5 mg SC/SL twice daily).

An **enlarging renal mass or obstruction may cause pain**. Because of impaired renal function, precautions must be taken when prescribing morphine or hydromorphone. Use lower doses, and if the dose is at its lowest limit change the dose frequency from 4 hs to 6 or 8 hs. Fentanyl is not metabolized or excreted by the kidney and may be preferable.

Prognosis measured in weeks prior to the onset of this problem (in addition to symptom control)
- Check **serum electrolytes, renal function, and FBC**.
- Collect **blood cultures if the person is febrile**.
- A **midstream urine sample** should be sent for microscopy and culture.
- Pass an **IDC** to measure residual urine and assess urine output regularly.
- **Plain pelvic X-rays** may display an obstructing calculus. Consider observation, lithotripsy, or removal using a Dormier basket.
- **Upper obstructions require discussions with a urologist and radiologist**.
- Use hyoscine butylbromide 20 mg SC and regular opioids and anti-inflammatories until the stone has passed.
- A **renal ultrasound** will show the level of obstruction in the upper collecting system.
- **In extrinsic compression, insertion of a ureteric stent may restore renal function**. If this is technically impossible, consider a percutaneous nephrostomy. It is imperative to warn the person that they may have an external drain for the remainder of their lives.
- **Lower obstructions may be relieved by passing an IDC** or **inserting a suprapubic catheter**. (It is unlikely that the catheter will be able to be removed again in this setting).
- **If febrile, initiate antibiotics after collection of blood and urine cultures**.
- **Ensure IV access for fluid hydration**.

Further reading
Oxford Textbook of Medicine, Vol. 3, pp. 249–250, 447.
Oxford Textbook of Palliative Medicine, pp. 310, 651.
Oxford Handbook of Palliative Care, pp. 324–327.

☼ **Urinary retention**

- This is a clinical diagnosis that is seen more commonly in men than in women.

Causes of acute urinary retention
Prostate disease (benign, malignant)
Infections
Neurological dysfunction
Medications (especially with anticholinergic effects which are cumulative)
Constipation
Post-operative (abdominal procedures)
Urethral strictures

History

People with acute retention of urine may present with suprapubic pain and inability to pass urine. They may have a history of increasing difficulty of initiating voiding that may be long-standing.

The history is different for people with chronic urinary retention, who typically do not have pain when unable to void but may have frequency or nocturia.

Physical examination

These people may be **distressed and are often hypertensive**. The **bladder is distended**, either palpable or percussable, and sometimes tender.

Investigations and management

Prognosis measured in hours to days prior to the onset of this problem (symptom control)

- **Administer analgesia and insert a urinary catheter**. If insertion of a urethral catheter is not possible, a suprapubic catheter may be necessary with specialist urological input.
- A person may have a **post-obstruction diuresis and may need gentle hydration to maintain comfort**.
- Be cautious about rapid decompression of the bladder, as there may be mucosal haemorrhage. Do not decompress at more than 500 ml/h.

Prognosis measured in weeks (in addition to symptom control)

- **This is predominantly a clinical diagnosis**. Occasionally **bladder ultrasound** may be necessary to establish residual bladder volumes.
- Additional investigations include **renal function tests and urine microscopy**.
- **Investigations must not take precedence over relief of retention**. After the catheter has been inserted, the cause of retention needs to be considered.

- Easily reversible causes (infection, constipation) may be addressed.
- More complicated causes of retention (medications that remain essential for this person, neurological causes, clot retention, pelvic tumours) may not be easily modified and these people may need the catheter to remain for the rest of their lives.

Prognosis measured in months to years prior to the onset of this problem (in addition to the above)

- **A urological consult will need to be sought** if a simple cause for urinary retention cannot be found.
- If people need long-term catheterization, it is preferable to consider a suprapubic catheter.

Further reading

Oxford Textbook of Medicine, Vol. 1, p. 879; Vol. 3, pp. 448, 450.
Oxford Textbook of Palliative Medicine, p. 649.
Oxford Handbook of Palliative Care, pp. 324–326.

☠ **Acute renal artery occlusion**

- This is a rare problem and may be difficult to diagnose because of the non-specific constellation of symptoms.
- Although it is not common, it is associated with significant morbidity.

Causes of renal artery occlusion
Atrial fibrillation
Malignancy
Vasculitis
Clotting disorders
Nephrotic syndrome

History
Acute onset of flank pain, fever, and haematuria without dysuria is typical. It is often mistaken for pyelonephritis, but, unlike infection, the fever will not respond to antibiotics. Occasionally, people may present with anuria, hypertension, altered mental state, and uraemia.

Physical examination
- People may have **renal angle tenderness on the affected side, fever, tachycardia, and hypertension**.
- An assessment of cognitive state is indicated as confusion can be caused by both malignant hypertension and uraemia.

Investigations and management
Prognosis measured in hours to days prior to the onset of this problem (symptom control)
Pain from an infarcted kidney may be unilateral or bilateral. The best option is fentanyl as it is not metabolized or excreted through the kidney. Low-dose morphine or hydromorphone may be used with extreme caution. It is advisable to start with low doses every 6 to 8 hs regularly rather than every 4 hs.

When bilateral damage has occurred, or there is unilateral damage in a person with previously limited renal reserve, **a person may become anuric and subsequently uraemic**. Control symptoms of uraemia such as itch, nausea, and twitching (p.184) as indicated.

Prognosis measured in weeks prior to the onset of this problem (in addition to symptom control)
- **Check FBC** (leukocytosis), **renal function** (hyperkalaemia, increased urea, and creatinine), and **coagulation studies** (coagulopathy). These are indicated, although in the early stages after the ischaemic event they may be within normal limits.
- **A raised LDH** may suggest embolic activity, but is non-specific.

- **Urine microscopy** may show haematuria and leukocytes, but with a negative Gram stain.
- **Doppler ultrasound** allows visualization of the renal blood supply.
- Other investigations (**angiography**) required to diagnose this problem are more invasive and may not contribute to a simple solution for this person.
- The choice of interventions depends upon the chronicity of the obstruction to renal blood flow.
- Unilateral damage to the kidney may not require intervention beyond pain relief and control of other symptoms.
- Bilateral damage may result in precipitous renal failure. An acute disruption to blood flow may respond to thrombolysis or vascular stenting. The benefit to the person will depend upon other comorbidities.
- A background of chronic narrowing of the renal artery with an acute insult is often a terminal event in this clinical setting. Dialysis is rarely indicated.
- Symptom control includes pain from renal infarcts and headaches from uncontrolled hypertension.

Prognosis measured in months to years prior to the onset of this problem (in addition to the above)

Investigations and management should include:
- **ECG** (effects of hyperkalaemia).
- **An IV pyelogram** will display no blood supply but does not differentiate between renal artery spasm, occlusion, avulsion, or an absent kidney.
- **Renal angiography** is the gold standard diagnostic test in people well enough to consider further therapy.

People with chronic renal artery stenosis and renal impairment may require dialysis prior to restoration of blood flow. Immediate restoration of blood flow to the kidney is the most important step in people with no long-term renal damage. Surgical bypass grafting may be considered in people who are functioning well where other therapies are not successful.

In the long term, people require management of hypertension and long-term aspirin. The cause of the obstruction defines other treatment.

People with underlying renal artery stenosis who progress to acute occlusion have a 4 year mortality of 50 per cent.

Further reading

Oxford Textbook of Medicine, Vol. 3, p. 258.
Oxford Handbook of Palliative Care, p. 322.

① **Renal vein thrombosis**

- This a difficult diagnosis to make, with gradual onset in most people.
- It can occur acutely, leading to renal failure.
- A renal vein thrombosis may propagate, leading to complications such as pulmonary emboli.

Causes of renal vein thrombosis
Nephrotic syndrome
Malignancy
Retroperitoneal fibrosis
Trauma

History

In the acute situation, people present with **flank pain, fevers** and **haematuria**. This may be associated with the complication of a pulmonary embolus. In severe cases with bilateral involvement, a person may present with anuria.

Physical examination

There may be a **low-grade fever and tenderness** over the **renal angle on the affected side**. The affected kidney may be ballotable.

Investigations and management

Prognosis measured in hours to days prior to onset of this problem (symptom control)

The symptomatic management is the same as for people with renal artery occlusion (p.296).

Prognosis measured in weeks prior to the onset of this problem (in addition to symptom control)

- Check **FBC, serum electrolytes, urea and creatine, LDH, and fibrinogen degradation products**.
- **Urine microscopy** will display haematuria and leukocytosis with no organisms evident.
- A **renal ultrasound and Doppler** is indicated to examine the size of the kidney and blood flow.
- Definite diagnosis is made by **selective venography, CT, or MRI**.
  These people should be **commenced on anticoagulation** with therapeutic doses of LMW heparin. This will need to be continued for the remainder of the person's life. Warfarin is not indicated.

Prognosis measured in months to years prior to the onset of this problem (in addition to the above)

- The initial management will depend upon the degree of venous occlusion.

- In bilateral thrombosis, a person may require dialysis.
- Usually, anticoagulation limits clot propagation, and renal function will return as clot is resorbed.
- In bilateral occlusion, or with pre-existing renal dysfunction, thrombectomy may be indicated.
- The prognosis of this condition is predominantly defined by complications such as pulmonary embolism.

Further reading

Oxford Textbook of Medicine, Vol. 3, pp. 228–229, 258, 328.

① **Genitourinary fistulae**

- A fistula is an abnormal connection between two hollow viscera or a hollow viscus and the skin.
- Abnormal communications may occur within the genitourinary tract or between the genitourinary tract and the GIT, blood vessels, the lymphatic system, or the skin. This section focuses on vesico-vaginal fistulae.

Causes of genitourinary fistulae
Cancer: local invasion
Cancer treatment (surgery, radiotherapy)
Local infections

History

The only history a woman may complain of is **fever and leakage of urine from the vagina**.

Physical examination

- **Physical examination may be unremarkable**.
- Often, there will be evidence of a frozen pelvis.
- Check for a **fever**.

Investigations and management

Prognosis measured in hours to days prior to the onset of this problem
- **This is a clinical diagnosis and no further investigations are indicated**.
- A person may be more comfortable with an **IDC**, which can divert the urine flow because of the larger bore of the urinary catheter lumen.
- **Continence pads** must be applied and changed regularly to maintain comfort and minimize the risk of excoriation.

Prognosis measured in weeks prior to the onset of this problem (in addition to symptom control)
It is unlikely that this group would be considered for surgical repair and therefore further investigations will not be of benefit. **An IDC** may **prompt closure**. Spontaneous closure is less likely to occur in people with a fistula occurring as part of a malignant process, and it is likely these people will be catheterized until their death.

Prognosis measured in months to years prior to the onset of this problem (in addition to above)
- **FBC, serum electrolytes, urea and creatinine**, and **urinalysis** are indicated.
- Further investigations include a cystoscopy or direct visualization of the vagina vault after the bladder has been filled with a dilute solution of methyl blue.

- In people who are considered for surgical repair, an intravenous pyelogram should be considered to visualize the patency of the upper urinary tract.
- A person who develops this problem as part of a complication of cancer treatment requires repeat staging investigations to exclude a recurrence of malignancy.
- Further treatment may be warranted in people who do not achieve spontaneous closure after insertion of an IDC. This will depend upon the cause of the fistula.
- Surgical correction may be possible in people without a malignant fistula.
- People with malignant fistulae may benefit most from a percutaneous nephrostomy.
- People who develop this problem after radiotherapy may require formation of an ileal conduit.

Further reading

Oxford Textbook of Palliative Medicine, pp. 263, 265, 655–656.
Oxford Handbook of Palliative Care, p. 91.

☼ Pelvic bleeding

- Bleeding may occur from the gynaecological, urological, or GIT viscera of the pelvis

---
Causes of genitourinary bleeding

Gynaecological cancers eroding major vessels

Fungating cancers of the vulva, vaginal vault, cervix, and endometrium

Bleeding from urological structures secondary to tumours, infections, calculus

Coagulopathy with pelvic pathology

Medications (anticoagulants, NSAIDS)

Cytotoxic agents (cyclophosphamide, ifosfamide)

History

- The initial step in the history is to **ascertain the origin of the blood loss**. It is sometimes difficult for people to ascertain whether blood loss is from the GIT or urogenital tract.
- Associated fever and dysuria suggest **infection**, which may be primary or occurring as a complication of obstruction.
- If bleeding is from the genital tract, other symptoms such as pain and offensive discharge must be sought.

Physical examination

- **Physical examination may be unremarkable**.
- Check for a **fever**.
- Check for evidence of **petechiae or bruising**.
- Percuss for a **tender and distended bladder**. This may represent clot retention.
- Do a pelvic examination to determine if there is local bleeding that may be amenable to local therapy.

Investigations and management

Prognosis measured in hours to days prior to the onset of this problem (symptom control)

When erosion of a major vessel has occurred, ensure that **crisis medications** (p.52) are available. These people should be nursed in a single room. Green or red towels help to minimize the visual distress of active bleeding. This is a clinical diagnosis and no further investigations are indicated. Discontinue any medications that may contribute to this problem.

- Genital tract bleeding:
  - These people may be frightened and anxious because of the ongoing blood loss. This may be an indication for sedation.

- Less torrential bleeding may be well palliated by packing of the vaginal vault with acetone-soaked sponges.
- Vulval bleeding may be managed with local pressure or epinephrine-soaked sponges.
- Comfort may be improved by insertion of an IDC.
- **Urological tract bleeding:**
  - Bleeding involving or proximal to the bladder may result in clot retention which should be considered if a person is uncomfortable and unable to pass urine. Even at the end-of-life, insertion of a three-way-catheter may allow the irrigated bladder to be cleared of clots. Continue regular irrigation to avoid further clots.

Prognosis measured in weeks prior to the onset of this problem (in addition to symptom control)

Collect serum electrolytes, urea and creatinine, FBC, and **coagulation studies**. Screen for bleeding complications such as **DIC** (p. 168).

- Genital tract bleeding:
  - Investigations to define the site of the bleeding should be undertaken. This may be by direct visualization by inspection of the external genitalia or a speculum examination. Further imaging with a **CT scan** may be necessary.
  - Commence **tranexamic acid** to help stabilize any clots that form.
  - If bleeding is from the vaginal vault, consult the gynaecological service for advice about how best to pack the vault.
  - Other options in this prognostic group include embolization of the artery supplying the bleeding site.
- Urinary tract bleeding:
  - Check urine microscopy and culture. Further investigations include **renal ultrasound** or CT scan to define likely bleeding sites.
  - Treat any infection and ensure adequate hydration.
  - In malignancy, a radiotherapy consultation should be considered.

Prognosis measured in months to years prior to the onset of this problem (in addition to the above)

- Transfuse if anaemic. Replace **platelets and FFP** if ongoing torrential bleeding.
- Ensure adequate intravenous access.
- Maintain blood pressure with adequate hydration.
- **Administer vitamin K 10 mg IV.**
- Consider the best imaging to define the source of bleeding, including selective angiography if the source of bleeding is not obvious.
- Genital tract bleeding:
  - Investigations and initial management should be simultaneously addressed. Seek urgent advice from the gynaecological team.
  - Treat pain, and nausea and vomiting as necessary.

- Urinary tract bleeding
  - Investigations and management should be simultaneously addressed. Seek urgent advice from urological services.
  - Organize an **urgent renal ultrasound and pelvic CT**.
  - Monitor for clot retention and organize insertion of a three-way catheter if this occurs.

Further reading

Oxford Textbook of Palliative Medicine, pp. 251, 653–654.
Oxford Handbook of Palliative Care, pp. 328–329

SNAP phase

1	Stable	All clients not classified as unstable, deteriorating, or terminal.
2	Unstable	The person experiences the development of a new problem or a rapid increase in the severity of existing problems, either of which require an urgent change in management or emergency treatment.
		The family/carers experience a sudden change in their situation requiring urgent intervention by members of the multidisciplinary team.
3	Deteriorating	The person experiences a gradual worsening of existing symptoms or the development of new but expected problems.
		The family/carers experience gradually worsening distress and other difficulties, including social and practical difficulties, as a result of the illness of the person.
4	Terminal	Death is likely in a matter of days and no acute intervention is planned or required.
5	Bereaved	Death of a patient has occurred and the carers are grieving.

From K Eagar *et al.* An Australian casemix classification for palliative care: technical development and results. *Pall Med* 2004; **18**: 217–226.

Australian-modified Karnofsky Performance Scale (AKPS)

Score	
100	Normal; no complaints; no evidence of disease
90	Able to carry on normal activity; minor signs or symptoms
80	Normal activity with effort; some signs or symptoms of disease
70	Cares for self; unable to carry on normal activity or to do active work
60	Requires occasional assistance but is able to care for most of own needs
50	Requires considerable assistance
40	In bed more than 50 per cent of the time
30	Almost completely bedfast
20	Totally bedfast and requiring extensive care
10	Comatose or barely rousable
0	Dead

From AP Abernethy et al. BMC Pall Care 2005; **4**: 7.

The LANSS pain scale: Leeds Assessment of Neuropathic Symptoms and Signs

A PAIN QUESTIONNAIRE

- Think about how your pain has felt over the last week
- Please say whether any of the descriptions match your pain exactly

1) **Does your pain feel like strange, unpleasant sensation on your skin? Words like prickling, tingling, pins and needles might describe these sensations**

   a) NO – My pain doesn't really feel like this .... (0)

   b) YES – I get these sensations quite a lot .... (5)

2) **Does your pain make the skin in the painful area look different from normal? Words like mottled or looking more red or pink might describe the appearance**

   a) NO – My pain doesn't affect the colour of my skin........................ (0)

   b) YES – I've noticed that the pain does make my skin look different from normal .... (5)

3) **Does your pain make the affected skin abnormally sensitive to touch? Getting unpleasant sensations when lightly stroking the skin, or getting pain when wearing tight clothes might describe the abnormal sensation**

   a) NO – My pain doesn't make my skin abnormally sensitive in that area... (0)

   b) YES – My skin seems abnormally sensitive to touch in that area............ (3)

4) **Does your pain come on suddenly and in bursts for no apparent reason when you're still? Words like electric shocks, jumping, and bursting describe these sensations**

   a) NO – I don't really get these sensations..................................... (0)

   b) YES – I get these sensations quite a lot...................................... (2)

5) **Does your pain feel as if the skin temperature in the painful area has changed abnormally? Words like hot and burning describe these sensations**

   a) NO – I don't really get these sensations..................................... (0)

   b) YES – I get these sensations quite a lot...................................... (1)

B SENSORY TESTING

Skin sensitivity can be examined by comparing the painful area with a contralateral or adjacent non-painful area for the presence of allodynia and an altered pin-prick threshold (PPT)

1) ALLODYNIA

Examine the response to lightly stroking cotton wool across the non-painful area and then the painful area. If normal sensations are experienced in the non-painful site, but pain or unpleasant sensations (tingling, nausea) are experienced in the painful area when stroking, allodynia is present

a) NO, normal sensations in both areas.. (0)

b) YES, allodynia in painful area only... (5)

2) ALTERED PIN-PRICK THRESHOLD

Determine the pin-prick threshold by comparing the response to a 23 gauge (blue) needle mounted inside a 2 ml syringe barrel placed gently on to the skin in a non-painful and then painful area

If a sharp pin-prick is felt in the non-painful area, but a different sensation is experienced in the painful area, e.g. none/blunt only (raised PPT) or a very painful sensation (lowered PPT), an altered PPT is present

If a pin-prick is not felt in either area, mount the syringe on to the needle to increase the weight and repeat

a) NO, equal sensation in both areas.. (0)

b) YES, altered PPT in painful area... (3)

SCORING

Add values in parentheses for sensory description and examination findings to obtain overall score

TOTAL SCORE (maximum 24)..

If score <12, neuropathic mechanisms are **unlikely** to be contributing to the patient's pain

If score ≥12, neuropathic mechanisms are **likely** to be contributing to the patient's pain.

From M. Bennett, *Pain* **92** 147–157, 2001.

Mini Mental Status Examination

The Mini Mental Status Examination is a quick way to evaluate cognitive function. It is often used to screen for dementia or monitor its progression.

Folstein Mini Mental Status Examination

Task	Instructions	Scoring	
Date orientation	'Tell me the date?' Ask for omitted items.	One point each for year, season, date, day of week, and month	5
Place orientation	'Where are you?' Ask for omitted items.	One point each for country, state, city, building, and floor or room	5
Register three objects	Name three objects slowly and clearly. Ask the patient to repeat them.	One point for each item correctly repeated	3
Serial sevens	Ask the patient to count backwards from 100 by 7. Stop after five answers. (Or ask them to spell 'world' backwards.)	One point for each correct answer (or letter)	5
Recall three objects	Ask the patient to recall the objects mentioned above.	One point for each item correctly remembered	3
Naming	Point to your watch and ask the patient 'What is this?' Repeat with a pencil.	One point for each correct answer	2
Repeating a phrase	Ask the patient to say 'no ifs, ands, or buts.'	One point if successful on first try	1
Verbal commands	Give the patient a plain piece of paper and say 'Take this paper in your right hand, fold it in half, and put it on the floor'.	One point for each correct action	3
Written commands	Show the patient a piece of paper with CLOSE YOUR EYES printed on it.	One point if the patient's eyes close	1
Writing	Ask the patient to write a sentence.	One point if sentence has a subject, a verb, and makes sense	1
Drawing	Ask the patient to copy a pair of intersecting pentagons onto a piece of paper.	One point if the figure has ten corners and two intersecting lines	1
Scoring	A score of 24 or above is considered normal.		30

Adapted from M.F. Folstein *et al.*, *Journal of Psychiatric Research* **12**,196–198, 1975.

Close your eyes

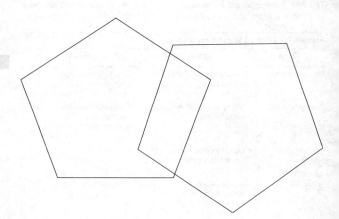

Glasgow coma score

The GCS is scored between 3 and 15, with 3 being the worst, and 15 the best. It is composed of three parameters; best eye response, best verbal response, and best motor response, as given below.

Best eye response (4)
1. No eye opening.
2. Eye opening to pain.
3. Eye opening to verbal command.
4. Eyes open spontaneously.

Best verbal response (5)
1. No verbal response.
2. Incomprehensible sounds.
3. Inappropriate words.
4. Confused.
5. Orientated.

Best motor response (6)
1. No motor response.
2. Extension to pain.
3. Flexion to pain.
4. Withdrawal from pain.
5. Localizing pain.
6. Obeys commands.

Note that the phrase 'GCS of 11' is essentially meaningless, and it is important to break the figure down into its components, such as E3V3M5 = GCS 11. A score of ≥13 correlates with a mild brain injury, 9–12 is a moderate injury, and 8 is a severe brain injury.

Source: G. Teasdale, and B. Jennett, *Lancet* **ii**, 81–83, 1974.

Index

H